WOMEN TAKE CARE

WOMEN TAKE CARE

GENDER, RACE, AND THE
CULTURE OF AIDS

KATIE HOGAN

CORNELL UNIVERSITY PRESS

ITHACA AND LONDON

First published 2001 by Cornell University Press
First printing, Cornell Paperbacks, 2001

Printed in the United States of America

Cornell University Press strives to use environmentally responsible suppliers and
materials to the fullest extent possible in the publishing of its books. Such materials
include vegetable-based, low-VOC inks and acid-free papers that are recycled, totally
chlorine-free, or partly composed of nonwood fibers. Books that bear the logo of the FSC
(Forest Stewardship Council) use paper taken from forests that have been inspected and
certified as meeting the highest standards for environmental and social responsibility. For
further information, visit our website at www.cornellpress.cornell.edu.

Library of Congress Cataloging-in-Publication Data

Hogan, Katie.
    Women Take Care : gender, race, and the culture of AIDS / Katie Hogan.
        p. cm.
    Includes bibliographical references and index.
    ISBN 0-8014-3627-3 (cloth : acid-free paper)–ISBN 0-8014-8753-6 (pbk. : acid-free paper)
        1. AIDS (Disease) in women. 2. AIDS (Disease)–Patients–Care–United States. 3. Sex
    discrimination against women–Health Aspects–United States. 4. Sex role. 5. AIDS
    (Disease) and the arts. I. Title.
RA644.A25 H64 2001
362.1'969792'0082—dc21

                                                                    00-012502

Cloth printing   10 9 8 7 6 5 4 3 2 1
Paperback printing   10 9 8 7 6 5 4 3 2 1

In memory of my sister, Mary,
1957–1994

CONTENTS

PREFACE

Within a nine-year period in the late 1980s and early 1990s, I lost my sister, her husband, and their two-year-old son to AIDS. Not long after, my fourteen-year-old niece, one of my sister's two surviving children, committed suicide. The circumstances surrounding their deaths have compelled me to write this book as a coping mechanism, a way of understanding. My sister, Mary, would have preferred that I drop out of graduate school and return to be with her in the small, lower-middle-class town where we both grew up. From Mary's perspective, such a move would have been far more helpful to her than what I was trying to do: survive the dual pressures of graduate school and AIDS through writing.

I realize that I cannot speak for my sister. My rendering of her views and experiences in these pages is no more fixed than my own writerly persona. But as a witness to some of my sister's experiences, I have come to see the themes of silence, representation, and HIV in a new light. What I saw Mary do in response to HIV was what I saw much AIDS literature and visual culture do: approach the topic by glorifying the elevated abstraction of the mother / good woman as a way of tempering the degraded meanings associated with HIV.[1] The problem with such a strategy is that it silences the lives of flesh-and-blood women and distorts the realities and struggles of those who have died.

For Mary, as for most women who have AIDS or are HIV positive, AIDS was just one of many difficulties. Owing to the many problems that had burdened us since childhood, my relationship with my sister was not ideal. Mary, a mother on welfare, was a high school dropout who felt deeply ashamed of this fact. In contrast, I was the only woman in my immediate family to seek out and piece together a formal education, and I stress "piece together" because I had numerous obstacles at every turn. When I received my undergraduate degree from an obscure state university near my home, Mary seemed both genuinely puzzled that I had managed to earn a degree at all and also deeply jealous. After I claimed a lesbian identity, she sometimes made homophobic and racist remarks about the women I dated or befriended. Part of her homophobia seemed to stem from her anger at her husband, who concealed his sexual relations with men; part of it also seemed to stem from her bitterness and jealousy over my modest achievements and the happiness I derived from them.

Despite the resentment and guilt I felt, which, from my perspective, ruined our relationship, Mary's experiences taught me how the stigma of AIDS brings into bold relief entrenched societal ideas about women and gender. My sister was obsessed with the various rumors that circulated in her community about how she and her husband, Jeff, contracted HIV. When the ambulance drivers who drove Jeff to the hospital (where he died two hours later) insinuated to her that he was a "junkie," Mary became infuriated with this stigmatized identity, but she didn't counter it with a true statement: "No, it wasn't drug use. Jeff had sex with men."

Mary responded to the multiple stigmas of her own diagnosis—stigmas that include engaging in gay sexual practices, belonging to a "minority" culture, injecting drugs, or having the visible signs of mortality—with fabrications. She told many people, including her two surviving children, nurses, doctors, caretakers, friends, and audiences who heard her lecture in schools and on the radio as a "woman living with AIDS," that she had contracted HIV through a blood transfusion. She hid the parts of her experience that conflicted with the injured, innocent image she fostered. My sister often constructed a representation of herself as benevolent, justifying her "lies" by evoking the cultural authority of her maternal work: she was protecting her two uninfected children. Mary tried to circumvent the stigma of AIDS by using the cultural symbols or rhetoric she thought would temper that stigma. She didn't want to feel blamed, and, I believe, she tried to challenge how the stigma of AIDS exacerbated her own internalized self-hatred. She died, however, still feeling ashamed that she had AIDS.

Some women—like my sister, an undereducated white woman—perform the roles of "good woman," "injured innocent victim," or someone who really doesn't *deserve* AIDS, as a strategy of self-protection against social rejection. I think my sister, wittingly or unwittingly, orchestrated this self-representation as a way to survive the stigma of AIDS in a culture in which women are still confined to the categories of good woman or bad. I am not saying that my sister was dishonest. What I am suggesting is that her self-presentation reveals how the languages of AIDS come laden with enormous prejudice, and that conventional ideas of women and the "maternal" offer a smooth way to alleviate the strain of this constricting prejudice. As I hope to show in this book, the strategy my sister used is common to much of AIDS writing and visual culture.

When I first began my research on women and AIDS-related writing, I naively thought the solution to the problem of American women and representations of the U.S. epidemic was visibility. Once women became visible in novels, films, magazine articles, and medical research, then the isolation I knew women felt, the isolation I felt as someone who was trying to write on women and AIDS, would vanish.

I soon discovered that the topic of women and AIDS—and, in turn, the topic of women and representation—is even more complex than I had first imagined. Literary and visual responses to the pandemic often embody troubling contradictions, and these contradictions suggest the effects of representation on women's lives. One of the central themes I explore in this book is how literary and visual responses to the pandemic, while breaking silence on women and AIDS, use traditional images of women to make the pandemic acceptable to white heterosexual Americans. In other words, while much AIDS-related writing and visual culture resists silence and invisibility, it also distorts and disguises women's experiences. Visibility alone does not guarantee a resonant cultural expression of women's experiences with HIV.[2]

I approach the topic of women, AIDS, and representation with a particular focus on the issue of care and the "good woman" figure. Such a focus is not meant to elide the caregiving work of gay men. Gay men continue to do enormous caregiving work in the AIDS epidemic, and are, in too many cases, taking the place of biological families who refuse to care for an ill family member. But gay men are often feminized, especially when performing work traditionally associated with women.

Furthermore, as Walt Odets discusses, uninfected gay men's excessive focus on loved ones or friends with AIDS is often interpreted as psychological distress caused by the epidemic.[3] Yet this same focus in women, HIV positive as well as negative, is often construed as appropriate. Furthermore, that gay men assume roles traditionally associated with women does little to challenge the historical association of women with nonpaid care.

In my own experience with my sister, for example, I was expected to assume the role of selfless, good woman in response to her situation. The message I got from Mary, my family, many friends, and from society—including graduate school culture—was that I should give up the unglamorous struggle of graduate school and move back home to take care of my sister. Since the serial deaths from AIDS in my family were already interfering with my emotional well-being and my education, why not just give up? If I wanted to be considered a good woman, this was the only option, even though my sister had ample caretakers, the quality of my relationship with her was very poor, and the impact of such a decision would probably have meant that I would now be either unemployed or underemployed.

While this issue of women, care, and AIDS is a crucial one for us in the United States, it is a crisis of catastrophic proportions in developing countries.[4] With more than thirteen million AIDS orphans predicted by the end of the first decade of the new century, and with high rates of infection in Africa, Asia, the Caribbean, and Latin America, it is clear that formal and informal care will be a major economic, social, and political problem around the world. As opposed to the United States and Europe, most developing countries cannot afford to glorify the good woman as the symbolic solution to the stigma of AIDS, although denial and stigma are often strong responses to the epidemic throughout the globe. Yet traditional ideas about women in the context of AIDS, namely, that women gain their identity through the sacrifices they make for others, link women in developing countries with those in developed countries. Gender inequality and poverty increase the risk of infection for women in the United States and Europe, just as they do for women in developing countries.

One HIV-positive AIDS educator from Zimbabwe refers to women's sexual subservience as an outcome of their traditional roles: "For women there is no sexuality, only fertility" (quoted in Schoofs, "Death and the

Second Sex," 71). One Zimbabwean man's response to his wife's lack of interest in sex further illustrates women's gender inequality: "A prostitute is 100 percent what I want. My wife is just for cooking and washing" (quoted in Schoofs, "Death and the Second Sex," 71). Male sexual privilege, gender inequality, and poverty play a determining role in women's risk and treatment across the globe, affecting the quality of health care they receive (if any) and how they are represented in visual and written discourse on AIDS.

ACKNOWLEDGMENTS

This book would never have seen print without the help of many colleagues, friends, and family. At Rutgers University, I thank Marcia Ian, who threw me a lifeline at a crucial moment in my career. Her personal courage, intellectual prowess, and emotional openness sustained me through the first writing of this book. I am forever grateful to her. I also thank Wesley Brown and Richard Miller. In addition, I am grateful to Donald Gibson, Michael McKeon, Carolyn Williams, Barry Qualls, and Ann Baynes Coiro, who went out of their way to support me in subtle and not so subtle ways. I also thank Dr. Monica Devanus of the Teaching Excellence Center for inviting me to teach in an interdisciplinary program on AIDS and the Women's Studies Program for supporting my course on women and AIDS.

At the City University of New York, I would first like to thank the Faculty Publications Program and its 1998–99 members, Frederick De Naples, Carlyle Thompson, Cheryl Fish, and most especially, Linda Grasso and Nora Eisenberg, for their careful reading of drafts and their unwavering faith in my ideas and writing. Members of the English Department at LaGuardia Community College, City University of New York, have also assisted in the completion of this book. First, I would like to thank my chair, Sandra Hanson, for her support, and my mentor, Phyllis Van Slyck, for her time and friendship. Gail Green-Anderson, Leonard Vogt, Tom Fink, Liza Fiol-Matta, and Adesimba Bashir also offered insightful commentary and encouragement. My thanks also to Catherine Costa of the English Department and to Lakshmi Bandlaumudi and Lorraine Cohen of the Social Sciences Department for providing feminist community.

I am grateful to the National Women's Studies Association and the Research Foundation of CUNY for validating the writing of this book through fellowships and grants and to Jeffrey Williams of *the minnesota review* for publishing my first essay on women, AIDS, and literature. A heartfelt thanks to Nancy Roth, Nan Bauer Maglin, Donna Perry, and Dana Heller for publishing subsequent work. At Cornell University Press, I thank my editor, Bernie Kendler, for his high standards and faith in me, and reviewer John Erni of the University of New Hampshire for his excellent feedback.

To members of my family, including my father and late mother, Andrew and Norma Hogan, my siblings Linda Gass, Debbie Carey, and Andy Hogan, and my nieces and nephews, Kaly, Sarah, Amy, Aran, and Jeremy, thank you for putting up with me. I also thank my late brother-in-law, Jeff Anderson, niece, Amanda Anderson, and sister, Mary Hogan Anderson, to whom this work is dedicated. To Norman Redlich, Gloria and Harold Redlich, Deb Redlich, Marcy Klein, and Nancy Redlich, thank you for supporting me in the very early stages of the project.

Because the impetus for this book stems from painful experiences, the research and writing were very difficult to do and took a long time. Rachel Stein, an ally and close friend, convinced me that no matter the obstacles, the book would get done. Her friendship and consistent loving support have been invaluable. Linda Grasso, who has been generous with her heart and time, has also supported me through the last two drafts of this book and spent many hours over two summers discussing the project. I would also like to thank Marion Banzhaf and Stephanie Hartman for their many helpful comments.

With the deepest passion and love, I thank most of all my life partner, Paula Martinac, who began to write at the age of seven and hasn't stopped. Your devotion to language, to clarity, and to the completion of projects, and your help in every aspect of the writing of this book, have forever changed my life. I am a better person and a better writer because of you. And to my puppy, Lucy, thanks for teaching me the importance of play.

WOMEN TAKE CARE

CHAPTER I

WOMEN AND AIDS

PARADOX OF VISIBILITY

> There has been no significant departure from the expectation that women will be the primary caregivers. Unshaken by numerous changes in public and work life, belief in women's primary responsibilities for home, family, and caring remains relatively resolute.
>
> Julia T. Wood, *Who Cares? Women, Care, and Culture*

The ancient idea of self-sacrifice and caretaking as woman's fate is a prevalent theme in many narratives on AIDS. Self-sacrificing mothers, caretaking sisters, nurselike lesbians, vigilant surrogate mothers, forgiving wives, and similar figures populate fiction, drama, film, television, and documentaries on the epidemic. This "good woman" generates not only compassion for people with AIDS but also nostalgia for women's traditional caregiving and self-sacrificing roles. As a result, AIDS literature and popular culture are paradoxically a place where the expression of feelings and sympathy for people with AIDS comfortably coexist with a subtle longing for idealized, nurturing women. I interpret this as part of a larger response to epidemics and to ideas about gender, illness, caretaking, and sacrifice, and examine how all of these are connected historically as well as in contemporary Western culture and literature.

Popular women's magazines routinely counter the antiquated image of the selfless woman with the popular image of the modern, independent woman who gets her needs met. A magazine such as *Self*, with its unrelenting focus on female professional individualism, argues that the angel in the house is dead and gone. But vestiges of the old model prevail.[1] Symbolic use of "woman" as self-sacrificing caretaker structures numerous representations of women, both past and present; these ideas are not obsolete, nor are they unique to representations of women in the AIDS epidemic.

Woman as caregiver has staying power in Western culture because she performs important cultural and physical work. Conceptualizing women as sacrificers and caregivers bolsters the historical association between care and the private realm of women and family. It says that caring for others is not the concern of public institutions or of private industry, even though the market value of informal caregivers' labor is estimated at $196 billion a year, compared with $32 billion for formal home health care and $83 billion for nursing home care (Levine; Arno, Levine, & Memmot). Yet numerous narratives replete with this caregiver image repeatedly construct the issue of care itself, a complex public issue, as a private, personal one that must be seen to by individuals and families. This notion also equates what counts as "good woman" with qualities such as selflessness and sacrifice—personal qualities that are devalued in the public sphere of work and politics, yet overwhelmingly expected of women.[2]

To idealize self-abnegation as womanliness glorifies a psychological stance that undermines women's ability to cultivate and practice agency. The physical, mental, and professional costs to women when they cast aside a self-created, dynamic identity in favor of responding to the needs of others in distress are concealed behind the loving spectacle of women's sacrifice. Yet most institutions in American society, including the family, the entertainment business, and the health-care industry, to name a few, acknowledge only the positive features of women's care and sacrifice, while strategically erasing the downside. And when women are constructed in contemporary representations as independent agents, they are often depicted as self-involved and heartless.[3]

Furthermore, idealized, selfless woman "costs" not only women as a group but potentially any person who is marginalized. Images of privileged sacrificial white women and girls function symbolically as the heterosexual feminine norm; they signify the ideal female citizen. That is, the culturally and historically entrenched mandate of good woman is a self-serving invention not only of dominant men but of dominant women as well, who often use the paradigm against less socially and economically privileged people. Language and culture surround women with an abundance of signification and ideas of womanliness; but the kinds of signification with which a woman figure is surrounded depend as much on race, class, and sexuality as on gender. This is a crucial insight that I develop in this book.

Clearly, AIDS is not the only lens through which to address the traditional paradigm of sacrificial care, but it is an extremely instructive lens. Epidemics require a tremendous caretaking response, just as desperately as they require medical research and treatment, and so it is fortuitous for society that many women enact the definition of good woman. But in the AIDS epidemic, which has always affected women, glorifying the equation of good woman with selfless care deflects attention away from diverse women's infected bodies and complex experiences. Even women who are infected construct themselves, or are constructed, in traditional terms, as caretakers and sympathizers rather than as sexual, flesh-and-blood people who are infected or at risk, a rhetorical practice I explore in Chapter 2.

In literary responses to AIDS, whether a fictional character is HIV positive or negative, her own health, sexuality, and personal history are rarely, if ever, developed and explored in their own right. For example, in Tony Kushner's *Angels in America,* women's sexual health is rendered irrelevant. It does not occur to critics how the character Harper Pitt, who is married to a closeted gay man, might be at risk for infection.[4] It is as if her position in the epidemic as something more than a victimized wife and fictional angel is unthinkable. The point is that the so-called counter AIDS narratives that set themselves up as exposing the "official" story are in fact part of the mechanism that obscures women's social realities.

Most important, the ideal of the nurturing woman makes "queer" Americans look good; yet again, in so doing, it presses women into conventional roles of mothers, caretakers, and wives.[5] Chaste images of women infuse respectability and female compassion into an otherwise shame-ridden and frightening discourse of queer sex, injection drug use, urban cultures, and poor developing countries ravaged by epidemic.[6] The kinds of images and identities linked with AIDS are not ones that dominant American society wants to associate with the nation; yet the epidemic must be discussed, and so the use of good woman, a use not unique to HIV, sanctions the discourse. Similar to medical and media representations, AIDS literature and popular culture often evoke traditional ideas of women to cultivate sympathy in readers and viewers while simultaneously reproducing the dominant power structure that says that good women are self-denying women who willingly care.

Throughout this book, I maintain that caretaking and sacrifice are fundamental human experiences, worthy of society's time and support, and that literary and visual responses to AIDS are forged to generate compassion and care. But it is worrisome that those members of American society who sacrifice the most are often those with the least amount of power, and this observation holds true in the age of AIDS as well.[7] It is also problematic that Western culture, history, myth, family, and economic structures continue to link caretaking activities with certain groups of people, mainly women, instead of viewing care as the responsibility of the entire society. As stated above, conceptualizing caretaking as female and equating self-sacrifice with "good woman" make it nearly impossible for many women to practice self-care. Women and minorities, who labor under the burden of being defined as the inevitable, biologically destined caretakers of the world, are often the last to receive care in the AIDS epidemic.

For example, a standard medical practice in the treatment of HIV has been to use the viral load measurements of men to determine whether or not an adult patient—regardless of sex or race—should begin taking protease inhibitors. Recent research suggests, however, that viral load in women's bodies is not equivalent to viral load in men's bodies, so that what appears to be an innocuous viral load in men is, when measured in women, a sign that the woman's immune system is seriously compromised and she should begin taking protease inhibitors (Bethea, 4). But because there has been a paucity of research on women and AIDS, basic understandings such as this one are only just emerging. Even more basic to the history of the epidemic is an accurate account of women and people of color in the official story of AIDS; this too has been a long time coming.

In 1997, AIDS was the third leading cause of death for women ages 25–44 in the United States, and since 1990 it has been the leading cause of death for African American women in the same age group. As of 1996, African American women composed 59 percent of all cases of women with AIDS; Latina women composed 19 percent.[8] Yet from 1996 to 1997 stories appeared in U.S. newspapers, magazines, and on television news programs jubilantly reporting the "end of AIDS." What was rarely mentioned in these accounts, including official announcements made by the U.S. Centers for Disease Control, was the 3 percent increase in deaths in women due to AIDS during the same period (Denison, "Women and AIDS," 4). Rebecca Denison, the founder and editor of *World*, a newsletter by and for women with HIV infection, reports that "women now account for 20% of new AIDS cases, compared to 18% in 1994, 13% in 1992 and 6% in 1982" ("Women and AIDS," 4). *New York Times* writer Sheryl Gay Stolberg has also challenged the widespread celebratory tone by pointing out that the 19 percent drop in deaths from AIDS attributed to the antiviral drugs known as protease inhibitors "has primarily benefited white men" (1).[9] Likewise, at the Third National Conference on Women and HIV in Pasadena, California, U.S. Representative Maxine Waters referred to "gaps in our progress. Not included in this success story are women and people of color" ("Determination").

Accompanying these gaps and omissions is the ubiquitous linking of women to sacrificial care in visual and print culture on AIDS. Perpetuation of this image suggests a deep investment in the paradigm of female sacrifice as biological fact, making representational issues of women and the epidemic far more complex than they may at first seem. By focusing on how particular texts and writers unwittingly reproduce a historically entrenched paradigm of sacrifice and care, and by pointing out how this same paradigm is deeply embroiled in narratives of race and sexuality, I am proposing that visual and print culture on the epidemic participates in a long-standing demand for female sacrifice at the same time that it challenges many aspects of the way the epidemic is conceptualized. Such a contradictory pattern highlights the tenacity of a traditional paradigm of women's sacrificial care, not the aesthetic or political failure of any particular cultural expression, writer, or representation.

Pointing out that popular literature and visual culture on AIDS activate an old-fashioned conception of sacrifice and caretaking, one that continually places women in the subordinate, sacrificer category, may seem heartless or a misconstruing of what is best in women's psychology and socialization. At the risk of seeming heartless, however, I want to insure for AIDS criticism what Dorothy Allison calls the ability to "read [texts] cynically" ("Question," 16). Cynical reading does not, as is so often argued, rule out inspired, deeply felt, passionate claims for the power of imagination, literary themes of hopefulness, and visions of social and political change (Rorty, A48). In critiquing AIDS culture from a "cynical," debunking perspective, I want to question the notion that since AIDS is so unambiguously devastating and rooted in the suffering body, the multifaceted AIDS communities of the world should just be grateful for whatever publishing—or any other corporate media venue, like Hollywood or the Broadway stage—has to give.

In text after text, the patriarchal paradigm of good woman governs the representation of women in the epidemic. The same brave, moving, well-constructed narratives of life during an epidemic may rely upon a conception of women that contributes to their subordination—in the epidemic and in society in general. In the AIDS fiction and popular culture considered here, texts reinscribe the idea of sacrificial good woman—turning women's bodies into a gendered icon, both textual and visual—even though these same texts also rigorously interrogate other cultural myths associated with the epidemic, such as that women do not contract HIV infection or that gay men are subhuman sexual predators who deserve to be punished.

Many women affected by HIV/AIDS might not care much about cultural ideas and representations of women—particularly literary representations. But representations are symbols, and language and symbols have an impact on women's material lives.[10] Coding AIDS as male and deviant, united with the historically entrenched notion of woman as "natural" caregiver, can act as an obstacle to women's health. For example, one mother with AIDS writes, "Women will care for children and partners with HIV and ignore themselves" (Siporen, 6). This sentiment is repeated over and over in the diverse discourse of women and AIDS. A recent publication of the New Jersey Women and AIDS Network lists women's socialization, which inclines them to put the needs of others before their own, as a *barrier* to women's health care. Women such as the one quoted above are not rejecting the human need to receive or give care; they are questioning the centuries-old idea that care and sacrifice are women's work alone.

While this book does not offer an answer to the question of caretaking, it is informed by answers other scholars have proposed. In *Who Cares? Women, Care, and Culture,* Julia T. Wood argues that the only way to change the paradigm of care that exists in Western culture is by ending its natural and inevitable association with women; by reframing care as a public, as opposed to a private, issue; and by devising a livable concept of individuality for women that truly acknowledges autonomy as well as interdependence. Neither idealizations of self-sacrificing women nor idealizations of individualism will save women from the fate of having to sacrifice themselves or solve the problem of care in American society.

Thus, my focus throughout this book is on AIDS narratives as discourses of women's caretaking and sacrifice, offering both traditional and innovative conceptions of women in the epidemic and exposing, often unwittingly, the issue of care and women as central in both AIDS and public life more generally. By zeroing in on the contradictions of these texts, and by exploring how they perform both progressively and conservatively, I will show that care, sacrifice, and women are hidden themes in progressive responses to the epidemic. In this way, representations of women and AIDS are paradoxes of visibility because women are present but only in terms of an ancient, sentimental conception of sacrifice and caretaking.

In developing this argument, I explore epidemics in Anglo-American literature in relation to nation building and conceptions of women; the rhetoric of the good-bad woman and the separate spheres, and the implications of this tradition for women in the age of AIDS; and the role of sentimentality in disseminating or promoting the legacy of the sacrificing woman. In the chapters that follow, I incorporate knowledge of the lived complexities of HIV-positive women and depart from the claim that women are invisible in the epidemic. Instead, I argue that women have always been visible in the AIDS epidemic, but in terms of a particular notion of what counts as "woman."[11] A critical examination of representations of women and AIDS suggests that breaking silence and smashing invisibility, although crucial, may not be enough.

Narratives of Epidemic, Narratives of the Nation

Narratives of epidemics within Anglo-American literature and popular culture comprise a mixture of outright denial and highly coded, metaphoric, oblique references. Joann Krieg attributes this long-standing cultural practice to the culture's roots in biblical tradition, obsessive nationalism, and literary romanticism. "The reasons for the denial and obfuscation have to do with national pride and economic fear," Krieg writes, as well as with preserving the Puritan view of America as "the New Jerusalem" (2, 4). Cultivating national pride and nationalism has always meant that a good citizen must be disease-free and orderly; and to maintain the view of

America as disease-free and orderly depends upon the circulation of dominant stories of diseased, chaotic Others as well as stories of good, clean citizens.

Literary documents of the fledging New World, such as Charles Brockden Brown's *Arthur Mervyn, or, Memoirs of the Year 1793* (1799–1800) and Nathaniel Hawthorne's "Lady Eleanor's Mantle" (1838), suggest that American writers often depicted Europe, with its old cities and alleged decadence, as a place of disease, both moral and physical. The New World was ideologically constructed as a place of redemption and as a space free of all of the problems of the Old, including the problems of space, dirt, political corruption, and disease. Situations and persons that challenged this evolving mythology had to be repressed or abstracted into cautionary tales and moral narratives. In cases in which this option was not possible— for example, in instances when the emergence of an epidemic could not be traced back to Europe, Asia, Africa, or Latin America—the blaming practices of Western culture sought out a New World scapegoat. Recent immigrants or any minority existing outside the dominant, white, male, Protestant majority were singled out as the source of infection. Epidemic illness became a metaphor for political anarchy and depravity within the nation. Debates within the emerging field of U.S. medicine simultaneously questioned and extended many of these scapegoating constructions and practices.

Not surprisingly, literary responses to epidemics reveal many of the same paradigms and debates occurring in society at large. If an epidemic disease was interpreted as threatening to the formation and independence of the nation, it was commonly treated in literary texts in a highly allegorical, indirect manner, and the origin of the disease was firmly located outside the boundaries of the New World. The impact of health epidemics on American writers has been, and remains, profound: "American writers were required either to ignore those aspects of American life that indicated a less than ideal environment, or to refer to them obliquely by resorting to analogous situations or topics" (Krieg, 4).

Recent social histories of illness, such as Sheila M. Rothman's *Living in the Shadow of Death: Tuberculosis and the Social Experience of Illness in American History*, point out the gap between literary narratives of illness and the physical deterioration, psychological pain, and societal responses that accompany disease (8). Rothman examines literary authors and writers of medical case studies who hide the true physical ravages of disease and suffering. Critics and social historians commonly read the absence of a graphic language of illness as an expression of basic human fear. The habit of "softening" the reader's and the writer's confrontation with death and disease is typically understood as a timeless human response to the fear of mortality (Krieg, 96). But there are additional meanings attached to literary and cultural renderings of epidemic death, as Krieg's focus on the relationship between U.S. nationalism and literary movements suggests.

The United States has a long tradition of distorting the nature of epidemics as it constructs narratives and moralities to justify power structures. Moral narratives that arise in times of epidemic regulate and subdue social outcasts in order to preserve dominant concepts, such as that the United States is an idealized, "clean" country and middle-class white women are good, asexual mothers. Epidemics offer opportunities for the solidification of social hierarchies that intersect with nationalism and deep-seated, unconscious psychological responses. Hawthorne's story, "Lady Eleanor's Mantle," is one of the few literary documents in existence that alludes to a 1721 smallpox epidemic in Boston. One reading might focus on the gap between the time of the epidemic, 1721, and the time of its transformation into a literary document, 1838. Krieg, for example, proposes that Hawthorne's decision to base his 1838 story on a 1721 smallpox epidemic suggests Hawthorne's own alternating denial of and fascination with several cholera epidemics that took place during his own time (9).

But what is significant about this story in terms of contemporary literary and visual representations of women and AIDS is Hawthorne's decision to transform the factual source of infection—allegedly sailors from the Old World—into a young, unmarried, haughty, British "Lady Eleanor," who arrives in Boston by ship to visit relatives. Hawthorne's story associates an attractive, upper-class British maiden with an epidemic that threatens the entire city of Boston. Lady Eleanor and her mantle—the vector of transmission, created by an elderly English woman as she was dying—infect almost all who attend a ball held in her honor. Here Hawthorne not only augments the alliance between disease and the decadent, aristocratic Old World; he contributes to the entrenched cultural mythology of woman as alluring, duplicitous infector. This archetype reappears in contemporary narratives on AIDS.

Bad woman images abound in popular science, mass market magazines, television programs, and medical research, treatment, education, and prevention practices (Kitzinger, 95–109).[12] In May 1983, the *Journal of the American Medical Association* unabashedly published an article with the woman-blaming title "Acquired Immunodeficiency with Reversed T4 / T6 Ratios in Infants Born to Promiscuous and Drug-Addicted Mothers" (Rubinstein, Arye, et al.). Here, woman is a pathological, irresponsible, hypersexual, diseased mother who infects her own helpless child. Tellingly, the mother's own health is erased by the title's focus on her "effect" on the child. In other words, Hawthorne's oblique treatment of the original 1721 Boston smallpox epidemic—his "mask[ing] . . . in metaphor" an actual reference to the 1721 event (Krieg, 105)—is just one of many noteworthy aspects of his contribution to traditional literary reactions to epidemic disease.

For example, in *Long Day's Journey into Night* (1956), Eugene O'Neill depicts a woman's indifferent and inept response to her son's struggle with tuberculosis. Her drug use is implicitly blamed for the breakdown of the family. O'Neill directly refers to an illness that he himself experienced rather than couching epidemic disease in the distant past, as did Hawthorne; and yet, as in Hawthorne, woman is the figure of blame. What these literary examples suggest is that writers, just like society at large, often react to the fear and mystification of epidemic disease by resorting to narratives of condemnation: women, blacks, Jews, immigrants, the poor, urban dwellers, and so on, are causes of misery.[13] When epidemics and people's experiences of them make their way into historical and literary texts, the perspectives of "outsiders" are rarely developed and dramatized (Krieg, 9).

But epidemics in the United States also generate narratives of racial and class superiority. In the nineteenth century, "spiritualizing" the ill person's body was a prevalent way for writers to acknowledge the disorder of epidemic disease without jeopardizing a morally robust national identity. The confluence of nineteenth-century New England transcendentalism with several widespread tuberculosis epidemics resulted in the cult of the etherealized/spiritualized literary body. Famous examples of literary bodies being "consumed" by "consumption," as tuberculosis was then called, include Harriet Beecher Stowe's Little Eva and Louisa May Alcott's Beth March. Because the model of illness consolidated in the pages of Stowe and Alcott, and in the letters, diaries, and everyday behavior of

New England men and women, was associated with white middle- and upper-class characters, tuberculosis became a poignant and fashionable disease, an index to one's sensitivity and refinement, in a way that epidemics such as yellow fever and cholera never did. Instead of a narrative of condemnation, tuberculosis offered, at least for a limited time, a narrative of superiority.

Yellow fever and cholera were linked to the poor, the immigrant, and the urban ghettos; these diseases moved quickly, bringing death within weeks or days, and were not as prone to extended literary dramatization. In contrast, tuberculosis "consumed" the body slowly, over many years, and could even be viewed as chronic, although it was almost always fatal. Manifest in the body of a white, upper-class Christian or child, consumption became a mark of superiority; in the bodies of the "outsiders," tuberculosis signified immorality and depravity, or, at the very least, "minority" status.

By the late nineteenth and early twentieth centuries, consumption's name had changed to tuberculosis (Krieg; Rothman). When the illness was associated with individuals society deemed citizens with rights, it was seen as "consuming" or refining the ill person's body; materialism was being replaced with pure spirit. The ill person was seen as having insight and sensitivity. As the victims of the illness changed from the middle and upper classes to the poor, the working classes, and immigrants—that is, to less than ideal citizens—it assumed negative signification. Thus its name changed from the more literary to the more medical. Now the disease was associated with drunkenness, poor hygiene, and other immoral behavior.

This nineteenth-century narrative strategy of etherealizing the "valuable" ill body appears in contemporary strategies on AIDS (Krieg, 146).[14] We are no more willing today than people were in the nineteenth century to address the full politics of the disease in a direct, graphic manner. In an effort to preserve a particular national image, now as then we employ the spiritualizing process, the replacing of materialism with spirit even though this strategy is not available to all who are ill. In particular, as I argue in Chapter 3, the white child's body is more likely to be etherealized than is the white upper- and middle-class woman's and man's body; and "woman" as naturalized caretaker and savior of the family and nation is also evident in both centuries' literary maneuvers.

Thus, as in past literary and cultural responses to epidemics, the disease itself is less important than the disease as an opportunity for consolidating certain national values and ideas. Literary or visual texts do not deny "true" pictures of physical disease; instead, they inspire, in an effort to create meaning and to control the image of the nation, what the epidemic means. Narratives of epidemic provide the opportunity to bolster or invent paradigms and ideologies. Even discourses that seem to speak openly and directly about epidemics, that rise above denial, use the fact of an epidemic to generate or revitalize ideas about what is a socially acceptable American, man, and woman.

From Jezebel to Florence Nightingale: Transforming Bad Women into Good

Woman as innately maternal and nurturing is often positioned as the opposite of woman as sexually alluring, predatory, diseased, and pathological, but the two ideas are actually interlocked. In the context of AIDS, women can easily switch from signifying moral elevation to signifying abjection. "Good woman" symbolizes all that is threatened—family, community, nation—by unclean, selfish people with the virus (Kitzinger, 95–109). If a woman is middle class and educated, she is seen as a passive, desexed victim who does not deserve to have AIDS—she is an "innocent bystander" (Kitzinger, 98). If a woman is a sex worker or some other socially unacceptable person, such as a "welfare mother," she becomes a mythological scapegoat and is blamed for passing HIV infection to men and their innocent wives and children. Unmarried women can easily be labeled "bad" just by the mere suggestion that they are sexually active.[15] But responding to the epidemic by placing the selfish "bad woman" in opposition to the idealized, caring "good woman" is an attempt to manage the category of "woman."

An example of gender and race as central ideas in the popular Anglo-American culture of epidemic is *Jezebel*, a 1938 "woman's" film starring Bette Davis and Henry Fonda. A yellow fever epidemic in New Orleans creates social, moral, and economic chaos, which serves as the impetus for the exploration of ideas about white southern womanhood and social constructions of race.

The yellow fever epidemic transforms Bette Davis's character from a dangerous southern "Jezebel" who rebels against societal expectations to a de-sexed, ministering angel.[16] In the first half of the film, Julie, played by Davis, commits several transgressions: she appears late at her own engagement party dressed in a close-fitting (masculine) riding outfit; and she wears a flamboyant red dress to the annual high-society Olympus Ball, an act of defiance that causes her fiancé, Preston, played by Henry Fonda, to break off their engagement, leave this wild southern woman, and head north.

Julie pays for her repeated transgressions by living in social isolation. No one wants to associate with a bad girl. A year later, she learns that Preston has returned to lead the community in its fight against the epidemic. Wearing a virginal lacy white dress, Julie humbly asks Preston to forgive her, only to learn that he has married a woman from New York State.

The yellow fever epidemic offers Julie an opportunity to redeem herself. Viewers see glimpses of ill, dying, and dead white males loaded on carts headed for "leper's island." When Preston falls ill, Julie devotes herself to him, even though he no longer loves her, and announces that, for the first time in her life, she is thinking of someone other than herself. She may die as a result of her work with the infected, but she is determined not to die a selfish, rebellious woman. The last image of Julie is of her riding in a wagon of dying men. Seated near her is a nun/nurse, symbolizing the kind of selfless, caretaking woman that Julie has now become. By the film's end, Julie is the self-abnegating, martyred woman Preston and society longed for.

One message of *Jezebel* is that the most significant aspect of any medical epidemic for women is that it offers them a chance to change, or, in some cases, to become even better than they already were. Those outside mainstream Anglo culture are denied this opportunity and denied representation of their physical health; their risk of epidemic infection is entirely omitted, assumed to be unspeakable. For example, the impact of the medical epidemic on the African American characters is unimportant in *Jezebel*. Instead, white fantasies of African Americans as childlike servants permeate the narrative. Julie's rebelliousness may render her an outcast in southern aristocratic circles, but her "happy darkies" adore and respect their mistress.

Jezebel teaches that in times of epidemic white women should use the crisis either to change from bad woman to good woman or to become even more self-sacrificing than they were before. Urging women to become even more concerned with family, friends, community, and nation at the expense of their own needs, health, and development is an underlying subtext of this, and many, epidemic narratives. Issues of women's health and the health of people of color are either transformed into narratives of morality or made incidental and ignored. The spectacle of Julie's conversion from bad woman to good woman drowns out her own risk of infection as well as the epidemic's impact on the enslaved Africans.

Barbara Hambly explores this racial aspect of the good woman by specifically focusing on the physical violence hidden behind the ideal. Like *Jezebel,* Hambly's 1998 novel, *Fever Season,* is based on a yellow fever epidemic in New Orleans, but Hambly's ideal female sacrificer is in reality a sadistic torturer of enslaved Africans. In the narrative, the community's investment in seeing the socially and economically powerful Madame Lalaurie as a beautiful, caretaking Florence Nightingale enables Lalaurie to wield power and mutilate and murder her slaves; the epidemic provides Madame Lalaurie with the caretaking opportunity she needs to perform the ideal, sacrificing female role. Always neat, clean, and composed, even after cleaning up the vomit of male yellow fever victims who die in her arms, Lalaurie exploits the paradigm as a way to hide her depraved torture of human beings. Thus, the same paradigm that mandates the angel in the house conceals unspeakable torture against those citizens it deems unfit to symbolize the angel-citizen or to benefit from her loving care. In Chapter 4, I explore in more detail the influence of the white sacrificial/suffering woman on representations of women who are not white or heterosexual.

The idea of "Julie transformed" continues in contemporary times in the film *Marvin's Room* (1996), a narrative that uses women's diseases and images of women's supposedly innate self-sacrifice as codes for gay men's experiences with AIDS. Sarah Schulman points out, "[A]s AIDS has become increasingly unpalatable as a subject for gay art, gay men have increasingly been moving to other diseases. Women with diseases have become metaphors for men" (71–72). *Marvin's Room* secures its own marketability in a homophobic culture by operating as a "woman's film" and by submerging a coded, gay narrative on AIDS in a nostalgic yearning for traditional, maternal femininity.

Adapted by Scott McPherson from his 1991 play of the same name, *Marvin's Room* is based on illness in the author's family as well as on his experiences as an HIV-positive gay man whose lover died of AIDS. McPherson himself died of AIDS in 1992.

Significantly, it is only when Lee, the main character in the film (played by Meryl Streep), gives up her aspiration to be a professional hairdresser and moves back home to caretake her senile, ailing father, disabled aunt, and unmarried sister do Lee's familial relationships with her sister and emotionally unstable son improve. Lee is a white, working-class, single, "bad" mother who is transformed into a noble, self-sacrificing, "good" mother by the film's end. Her withdrawal from professional training and waged work to manage her family members' health is considered irrelevant. The film never addresses how Lee can economically afford to give up her livelihood and caretake without pay.

No matter what her ambitions or economic difficulties, Lee is depicted as a selfish, unfeeling woman. She is the bad mother, sister, and daughter who has rejected her true role. In contrast, Bessie (played by Diane Keaton) is the good sister because she has stayed home to take care of their father and aunt for over twenty years. One of the key lines in the film underscores this view by stressing the differences between Lee and Bessie: "How can one sister be so good and the other so bad?"

Some enlightened reviewers have specifically commented on Lee's character: "*Marvin's Room* celebrates the breaking of a woman's will, when will is just about all she has" (Corliss); "My recommendation is: go see this one for the acting, but don't let your feminist guard down and be taken in by the essentially traditional ideology of women's lives the film seems to be peddling" (Lopez McAllister). However, most film reviewers are oblivious to the film's reactionary conception of self-sacrifice and care as women's work and of working-class women's lives. One reviewer describes Bessie as a radiant "devoted spinster" and "old maid" who "doesn't seem to mourn the absence of marriage and independence" (Guthmann, D3). Lee, on the other hand, is described as "the bad sister" and "family black sheep" who has refused caretaking duties (Guthmann, D3). Lee is "a bundle of anger and frustration whose idea of fulfillment is a cosmetology school diploma" (Shulgasser, C3). According to Janet Maslin, Lee is a "willful, selfish mother" ("Bittersweet Lessons," C15).

Film critic Roger Ebert celebrates *Marvin's Room*'s focus on "the healing power of sacrifice"; however, he, too, seems unconcerned with the way the film romanticizes the costs of the good woman role for Lee. Like

McPherson, Ebert does not consider how a naive view of the ethic of fe-male self-sacrifice tells women that they should forget about their own needs and predicaments and minister to their families. In this way, *Marvin's Room* solidifies the identification of "good woman" with natural caretaker at the same time that it uses this feminine ideology as a coded narrative about gay men's caretaking in the time of AIDS. Such con-structions of women in the context of family illness reinforce the message that women should do the work that society won't do. Once again, the linkage of "good woman" with care is naturalized, strengthened, and promoted as women's "true" work, even for HIV-positive women and women living with AIDS.[17] Caring, sacrificial woman emerges as the im-plicit paradigm, even in a "coded" AIDS discourse such as *Marvin's Room*, because the difficult issues of caring for others—money, power, culture, language, gender, race, and tradition—must be obscured for the sake of the nation.

Separate Spheres, Sacrificial Women, and AIDS

The transformation of Lee in *Marvin's Room* from bad woman to good has its roots in the concept of the separate spheres. In late-eighteenth-century England, the image of woman as sexually willful and dangerously corporeal was in the process of transforming into the nineteenth-century "angel in the house," a gendered figure that idealized a disembodied, self-less, pure womanhood. This does not mean that the dangerously corporeal image of woman vanished, but that this conception was subsumed under the more dominant idea of woman as angelic. As Mary Poovey points out, "In the process, woman became not some errant part of man, but his op-posite, his moral hope and spiritual guide" (10). Similarly, in nineteenth-century Anglo-America, sentimentality in domestic fiction constructed and celebrated the angel-in-the-house role for women. As I discuss in Chapter 2, Harriet Beecher Stowe's *Uncle Tom's Cabin* successfully em-ployed the associations of femininity, caretaking, nurturing, mothering, and women's "innate" morality to persuade white female readers to sup-port the abolitionist movement and put an end to slavery. Stowe's plot turns on the separation of mother and child, a device that highlights the quiet yet strategic transmutation of large-scale social problems into a story of individual heartache (Cvetkovich, 127).

At the end of the nineteenth century, even "deviant" women could gain entry into the club of good womanhood by demonstrating their innate inclination for service and morally inspired social change. Lesbians, as Lillian Faderman has argued, gained prominence "because what they did could often be seen as housekeeping on a large scale—teaching, nurturing, healing—domestic duties brought into the public sphere" (*Odd Girls,* 23). Thus, sentimental elements such as homeplaces, emotion, and mothering appear to be located within the confines of the private sphere, but they actually operate as a public discourse about women.

For decades, feminist literary critics and historians of women's history have debated how to interpret nineteenth-century women's relationship to this cultural imposition of separate spheres, with one camp arguing that it gave white, middle-class women access to the public sphere, an access that eventually led to social advocacy for women's rights. Other critics and historians acknowledge women's clever manipulation of the rhetoric of women's innate nurturing to further their own political and social agenda, but they argue that these skills did not, and still do not, eradicate the underlying private/public, Madonna/whore dichotomies that either render women invisible or turn them into mythological symbols. My purpose is not to resolve this debate. It is to show how the debate itself, and the ideology of separate spheres that we associate with it, still structure discourse in American culture, particularly the discourse on epidemics and caretaking. The sentimental metaphor of the separate spheres is central in understanding representations of women and AIDS.

Emotionality, femininity, relationality, and biological processes such as birth, illness, sexuality, and death are intertwined with separate spheres. In the nineteenth century, the separate spheres ideology attributed greater moral character to women, especially women who were also mothers. Women's involvement against child labor, in the temperance movement, in the abolitionist cause, and in women's suffrage was deemed women's maternal work, their caretaking of the nation. Ralph Waldo Emerson showed his support for women's suffrage in 1855 when he said, "Women are the civilizers of mankind. What is civilization? I answer, the power of good women" (quoted in Brownmiller, 162).

Carroll Smith-Rosenberg interprets women's purported moral superiority, and thus separation from the male-dominated public sphere, in still more positive terms. Smith-Rosenberg focuses less on how women used the moral superiority of their relegated position to subtly influence political and social change than on how women used this imposed (and often self-imposed) separation to build a women's culture. Products of women's separate culture range from published domestic treatises, fiction, poetry, quilting, and cookbooks, to lifelong, intense, "romantic" friendships. In fact, women's romantic friendships were often more erotically charged than were women's relationships with their husbands. As men located the meaning of social identity outside of the home, women supported one another and provided tenderness and companionship through courtship, marriage, childbirth, sickness, and death. Rather than seeing these women as pathetic victims and second-class citizens, or as liberal do-gooders who naively tried to make the world a better place, Smith-Rosenberg interprets these women as transgressive.

Woman as naturalized caregiver is inextricably linked to the invention of the public and private spheres. The metaphor of the private sphere harks back to ancient Greece, where, as Julia T. Wood notes, "life [was] divided into public and private spheres, men and women [were] placed respectively within them, and different values [were] assigned to each, the public being the more important in the life of a culture" (14). Separate spheres ideology permeates almost all aspects of the AIDS pandemic. It has coded AIDS as a male disease and as a "public," global crisis, while AIDS in women, as well as women's caregiving in response to AIDS, is still seen as a marginal, "domestic" problem. It contributes to the conservative image of woman as inevitable caregiver and moral teacher. AIDS discourse reproduces this traditional position of women because the separate spheres metaphor continues to shape U.S. culture at large.

In her essay "Separate Spheres, Female Worlds, Woman's Place: The Rhetoric of Women's History," Linda K. Kerber insists that "separate spheres" ideology is neither a relic from the past nor an ideology unthinkable in these postmodern times:

> For all our vaunted modernity, for all that men's "spheres" and women's "spheres" now overlap, vast areas of our experience and our consciousness do not overlap. The boundaries may be fuzzier, but our private spaces and

our public spaces are still in many important senses gendered. The reconstruction of gender relations, and of the spaces that men and women claim,
is one of the most compelling contemporary social tasks. (62)

Nowhere are Kerber's insights more applicable than in the case of
women and AIDS. The image of woman produced by the ideology of separate spheres does more than limit women's intellectual and emotional development and expressions; it also elides the complexities of women's corporeality.[18] In the context of AIDS, the "separate spheres" ideology hides
the fact that women contract AIDS, have contracted AIDS, and have died
of AIDS since the inception of the pandemic. Separate spheres ideology
continues to structure gender relations in such a way that the language of
AIDS is itself a gendered language, minimizing women's HIV infections
on the one hand, and contributing to historically entrenched sentimental
images of women as nurturers and ministering angels on the other. Furthermore, although separate spheres is rooted in a rhetoric of biology, nature, and instinct, this does not translate into a genuine concern for or complex engagement with women's health. Women are reduced to their
bodies in the sense that they are constructed as "natural" caretakers, reproductive vessels, or prostitutes who pass the virus on to babies or other
innocent victims. Yet this biological reductionism does not translate into
an interest in or knowledge of the impact of HIV on women. As Marcia Ian
argues, "biology is used to idealize women" once again. The notion of
women as natural caretakers, coupled with a nostalgia for a feminized domestic past, obscures women's corporeality.

The assumption that woman is a moral center devoted to the needs of
others is based upon the alienation of women from their bodies, since a
"true woman" requires a spiritualized, disembodied self-presentation. Yet
estrangement from their bodies contributes to women's passivity in sexual encounters, which in turn increases their risk of HIV infection. The
nineteenth-century Anglo-American "cult of true womanhood" demanded that "good" women be ignorant of their health and sexuality—a
view that is implicitly repeated in the desexed images and visions of
women found in contemporary AIDS literature and popular culture.[19]

The association between female disembodiment and enforced, dominant femininity remains a pivotal issue. Janet Holland, Caroline Ramazanoglu, Sue Scott, and Rachel Thomson have conducted research on

young women and safer sex practices that suggests that the etherealized, white, female body continues to control what counts as acceptable femininity, thus directing young women to estrange themselves from their bodies and desires (61–79). Not only does the disembodied angel in the house continue to shape what counts as (white) femininity, but this notion of femininity, because it discourages knowledge of sexuality and health, is precisely what puts young women's bodies at risk of HIV infection. Holland et al. found that although young heterosexual women are preoccupied with constructing an alluring "surface" sexuality in connection with a dominant femininity, this focus on physical appearance does not translate into an awareness of their sexuality or health. Young women know how to *appear* sexual and desirable for men, but they don't know how to feel comfortable about their sexuality or their bodies.

Women's risk of HIV infection, and more broadly the ways in which living in an age of pandemic jeopardizes all women's individuality and health, are hidden behind the nostalgic, entrenched rhetoric of separate spheres. On the most concrete level, this discourse impedes women's ability to gain access to AIDS education, treatment, and experimental clinical trials. As Carol Keeley explains, "Women are still dying sooner after diagnosis than men because the average physician can't accept that women are at risk of infection and so misdiagnose their condition, delaying treatment" (50). It is not that women are "trapped" by their bodies; rather, the impact of HIV on their bodies is ignored or transformed into moral narratives. For the average physician to "accept" that women are at risk would require him or her to rethink the cultural category of "good woman." Thus, women are reduced to their bodies' reproductive capacities and disorders and yet are never really perceived as bodies with health needs.

All in all, the cultural construction of women as biologically destined to care contributes to the conceptualization that AIDS is a male disease and that women's fundamental position in the pandemic is to take care of other people: to be their moral compass, to encourage others to respond to the afflicted with compassion, and to care for the physically ill. Women routinely acquire visibility solely in terms of their relationship to others; their identities are merged with their response to the physical and emotional needs of other people—partners, spouses, children, community, nation.

Women are taught to do what a culture wants them to do, just as they are taught to think that what the dominant culture wants is what they want (Wood, 33–61).

Claudia Koonz argues in *Mothers in the Fatherland: Women, the Family and Nazi Politics* that a majority of German women welcomed the gender and racial stereotypes disseminated by the Third Reich because these notions elevated motherhood and sent women back to the home, where they were protected from harsh working environments and low pay. The Nazi state mandated that women were not suited for the public sphere, and so domesticity became a space that was itself an extension of Nazi propaganda and infused with the nostalgia of sentimental female imagery. Women were expected to reproduce, to be nurturing mothers and practicing Christians, and most German women carried out these orders with vigilance and obedience. At the same time that Germany was celebrating motherhood, kitchen, and church, it was also committing mass murders against mothers, children, and families that it deemed subhuman.

I am not suggesting, of course, that the contemporary iconography of nurturing femininity in the discourses on AIDS, liberal as well as conservative, is being deployed to deflect attention away from state-sanctioned mass murder or to rationalize genocide. Nevertheless, Koonz's work suggests how the rhetoric of separate spheres, domesticity, traditional family values, and Christianity circulates as part of a larger state ideology. The symbol of woman as home is similarly being manipulated in the public sphere as a form of social control over women and all HIV-infected people.

HIV narratives become a way to perpetuate and affirm the historical practice of compelling those with lesser social status to be the quiet helpers; they will be morally and physically responsible for the caregiving work that Western culture devalues and refuses to validate through wages and recognition precisely because it is deemed "women's work" (Wood, 113–30). Women who challenge dominant—and dominating—concepts such as that they should subordinate their own needs, health, and development for the sake of others are labeled unfeeling. The mere questioning of the historical linkage of care, low value, and "good woman" can result in the accusation that one is "unfeminine," or, like the character of Lee, a bad mother and sister.

Feminist Theories of Sentimentality

Separate spheres and discourses of nurturance and care often overlap with sentimental rhetoric, a rhetoric that invokes the authority of human emotion and the body. Sentimentality is neither inherently pernicious nor empowering for women or other socially marginalized groups.[20] As Stephanie Smith argues, "The issue . . . is not whether sentimentality is 'good' or 'bad' but rather how it is used" (42). In the context of HIV/AIDS, however, sentimental rhetoric is a structure that conceals the psychic and physical violence of idealized assumptions of women's sacrificial caretaking. It disseminates conceptions of women's sacrifice and caretaking as always desirable, virtuous, and noble by constructing traditional roles as natural and by romanticizing the servile image of woman. It also implicitly constructs a discourse of race that divides women into desexed "good" and hypersexed "bad," for example, into Mammy (in the case of African American women) and Jezebel. Thus, it is crucial for women writers and feminist critics to challenge the patriarchal notion of sentimentality as pejorative, but the intersection of sentimental rhetoric, women, race, and AIDS suggests how sentimental representations have serious limitations. Feminist celebrations of the culture of sentiment look very different when viewed from the complex perspective of AIDS. Rather than persuading feminist critics to applaud the "cultural work" of sentimental representations, as such critics as Jane Tompkins encourage, my project argues for a more modulated approach, one that directly acknowledges the potential of sentimental rhetoric to facilitate the subordination of women.

Cathy N. Davidson warns that anyone "encountering [sentimentality] must be aware of its particular history in American literary history" (788). In nineteenth-century American literature and popular culture, sentimentality was associated with exaggerated emotionality, tearful women, and inferior writing and art. Linking sentimentality with women has been a way to keep women writers out of literary circles and professions for at least two centuries, if not more. Pejorative ideas about women and sentimentality have often reflected male writers and critics' fears of that "d——d mob of scribbling women," as Hawthorne referred to his female competitors. As Davidson explains, all nineteenth-century women, regardless of what they actually wrote, were dismissed as sentimental hacks, "while virtually no novels written by men have been given this derogatory label" (788).

Linda Wagner-Martin similarly argues that this long-standing use of the term as a denunciation of women's writing continued in the widespread trivialization of women's writing in the twentieth century. In the 1970s, women's autobiographical writing was dismissed as sentimental, while men's writing on their fathers was considered brave and innovative (95). In "Erotic Self-Images in the Gay Male AIDS Melodrama," Thomas Waugh refers to "our culture's put-down of forms too closely allied to bodily responses, like horror, arousal, belly-laughs, and weeping" (123). Reviewers in the *New York Times Book Review* frequently judge a given author's handling of sentimentality.[21] If a book is deemed worthy, it eschews sentimentality; if it is deemed unworthy, it is enmeshed in sentimentality's cheap web.

Ironically, one of the first feminist critics to approach the subject of nineteenth-century U.S. women's sentimentality is the antisentimentalist Ann Douglas. Douglas's main argument is that sentimental rhetoric is problematic because of its role in the commercialization of American culture and its dangerous anti-intellectualism. She explores how disempowered middle-class white women and male clergy transformed their marginal position into a powerful subcultural practice that fit in nicely with the aims and values of burgeoning consumer capitalism. For Douglas, the result was that capitalist materialism encased in sentimental rhetoric thwarted the intellectual promise of the nation more than any other element of the nineteenth century. For example, Douglas analyzes how the operations of sentimentalism and the emerging field of advertising are both about exercising "influence" over people's minds and lives. In sentimental culture, women and clergy direct their gentle "influence" toward the unconverted. Similarly, advertising functions by prodding the consumer to purchase a product unconsciously.

Douglas's reasons for denouncing sentimentalism sometimes seem elitist (her concern over the consequences of sentimental "spread" seems limited to its effects on literary intellectuals and elite intellectual movements), and her characterizations of Margaret Fuller and Herman Melville as victims of sentimental culture engage the very sentimental values her book denounces. Nevertheless, Douglas initiated the widely held view that sentimental rhetoric comprises a powerful ideology that permeates U.S. culture. As a result, it is Douglas's pointed critique of sentimentality that led to pro-sentimental critical texts by such scholars as Nina Baym and Jane Tompkins, who also agree that sentimentality is a broad, cultural category. Baym's and Tompkins's critical responses to Douglas are now considered standard feminist interpretations of women's sentimental texts.

Feminist critics widely embrace Tompkins's argument that sentimental domestic fiction suggests how the moral authority of women's domestic sphere influenced the public sphere of men and politics and thus crossed the boundaries of gendered spaces. In analysis of domestic fiction, one key argument is that sentimental texts are a covert attack on demented, patriarchal values. Nineteenth-century women writers fought the gender politics of literary reviews and canon formation by strategically appropriating the terms and values used to belittle and oppress them. In this way, women's sentimental culture figured as formidable anti-elitist interventions into the dehumanizing world of patriarchal capitalism, while being rooted in women's kitchens, parlors, gardens, and books. For example, in Harriet Beecher Stowe's *Uncle Tom's Cabin*, the author sarcastically uses the phrase "womanish sentimentalist" to indicate her awareness of the literary establishment's discomfort with the kind of novel she is writing (342).

Prior to Baym and Tompkins, texts associated with women or with "femininity" were either ignored or dismissed as commercialized, mass audience "trash" by both male and female critics. Most literary historians pigeonholed Stowe, Louisa May Alcott, and other popular women writers as "minor" and unimportant, a response that Tompkins challenges in her well-known 1985 study, *Sensational Designs*. Tompkins's book not only uses feminist literary criticism to challenge the gender politics of canon formation, but uses historical and political contexts as the key to understanding these denigrated texts. For Tompkins, the most important question one must ask is: What kind of cultural work does a sentimental text perform? Tompkins uses this framework to argue that Stowe's *Uncle Tom's Cabin* was a great piece of American literature even though literary critics dismissed the novel for years as "popular," "maudlin," and lacking in literary skill. Tompkins reads Stowe's influential narrative as possessing a uniquely feminine "sentimental power" and argues that nineteenth-century sentimentality "reorganize[d] culture from the woman's point of view," thus serving as the basis of the future women's liberation movement (124). In fact, Tompkins demonstrates how the novel's sentimental power challenged slavery.

The interrelated genres of sentimental melodrama, romance fiction, and women's "weepies" were of great interest to feminist literary and film critics in the late 1970s and early 1980s, the time when Tompkins and Nina Baym were reclaiming and rediscovering women's texts and lives. The Feminist Press reissued Susan Warner's *The Wide, Wide World* and Tompkins wrote the afterword; other writers, such as Fanny Fern and Louisa May Alcott, were the focus of much feminist scholarly activity. In 1982, Tania Modleski's application of feminist theory to the interpretation of romance fiction, gothic novels, and soap opera opened up an avalanche of cultural criticism on popular culture from an explicitly feminist perspective. In feminist film theory, many critics were questioning Laura Mulvey's theory of the male gaze by exploring the possibility of a female gaze or female spectator position.

In the early 1990s, Shirley Samuels broadened the discussion of feminism and sentimentality even further by editing a collection that reads sentimentality from a number of new perspectives. The overall theme of *The Culture of Sentiment* is that sentimentality is a complex aesthetic, cultural, and language-oriented practice that requires careful, theoretically informed analysis. Armed with critical perspectives such as poststructuralism, Marxism, new historicism, and African American criticism and theory, Samuels's anthology exploded the ingrained prejudice that sentimentality is a one-dimensional, simpleminded, middle-class woman's practice. One of Samuels's contributors, Lynn Wardley, argues that the sentimental genre is a cross-cultural genre with roots in West African spiritual practices (203–20).

Feminist literary critics continue to see women's sentimental and popular writing as intertwined with women's films, television programs, and other examples of popular culture. The gender politics involved in both the production and critique of texts labeled "sentimental" (e.g., soap operas, love stories, domestic narratives) continue to be scrutinized today in the field of cultural studies. Although contemporary feminist scholarship on sentimental aesthetic practice has become more critically engaged and less celebratory than scholarship of the late seventies and early eighties, it maintains its original position that revisionary understandings of women's writing and experiences under patriarchy are central to feminist criticism. Despite innovations, complexities, and advanced theoretical understandings of sentimentality, including Wardley's argument about the African origins of the culture of sentiment, sentimental texts—whether visual or written—still tend explicitly to favor the experiences of white, middle- and upper-class women. They also do little to dismantle the naturalized equation of good women and sacrificial care. The result is that these texts aggressively construct and produce "woman" and maternal femininity as decidedly white, middle class, and normative.

In opposition to these critical views, several literary critics, for example, Hazel Carby and Harryette Mullen, have extended and challenged the work of Tompkins and others in order to expose the "whiteness" of sentimentality. They show how black women writers, who had no choice but to employ a "white" rhetoric, did so strategically. Carby and Mullen document how black women writers negotiate sentimentality in such works as *Iola Leroy* and *Incidents in the Life of a Slave Girl*. Rather than being silenced by the inevitable conflicts they felt in using a white, middle-class-based rhetoric to describe black female experiences in a racist society, black women writers used the incongruity between their lives and this dominant discourse to expose the brutality of the supposedly superior white race.

Furthermore, feminist historians, including Linda K. Kerber, argue that women's sentimental culture addressed the aspirations only of white middle-class women, thus erasing altogether the experiences of poor women, immigrant women, and women of color. Kerber interprets sentimental conceptions of separate spheres ideology as a mechanism for middle-class consolidation, and she suggests that a feminist fascination with the metaphor of separate spheres shifts attention away from class and race issues.

However, as previously mentioned, Lynn Wardley argues in "Relic, Fetish, Femmage: The Aesthetics of Sentiment in the Work of Stowe" that the emotionality expressed in such sentimental icons as *Uncle Tom's Cabin* draws not upon Anglo-American middle-class culture, but upon the beliefs and practices of West African spirituality. Wardley's essay offers an expansive and hybrid definition of sentimentality, but she does not address the limitations, troublesome legacies, or multiple contexts in which sentimentality can be used.

Wardley argues for the "bodily nature of the sentimental genre and the genre's connection to women," viewing it as a genre of women's "physical labor of reproduction, sickness, and death" (206). But Wardley also mentions, although without elaboration, how "a feminized sentimentalism is also linked to the 'sivilizing' work of socialization" (206). It is precisely this "sivilizing" work associated with women that leads to the view of women's bodies as symbols of disembodied moral elevation and pedantic instruction.

On the whole, sentimental discourses and separate spheres assign women to the work of acting as moral symbols, a particularly pernicious construction in today's discourse on women and AIDS. While feminist literary criticism may perform transgressively in the context of academic culture, where books and articles that reclaim noncanonical perspectives and writers are perceived as a challenge to the professional status quo, on the whole, sentimental rhetoric is not necessarily transgressive or subversive, at least in terms of AIDS and traditional ideas of female self-sacrifice. The culture of sentiment potentially gives a "feminine" voice to the enormous suffering caused by the pandemic, but such representations also come with conservative ideas about women.

The problem with sentimental representations of AIDS lies not in their lack of skill or literary merit but in their uneasy fusion with a conservative domestic ideology. I view sentimental texts not as powerless and operating in a narrow, separate sphere but as a central, dominant ideology with potentially far-reaching effects on people's lives.[22] Douglas and Tompkins seem limited in their theories of sentimentality: for Tompkins, women's sentimental culture exposes the narrowness of literary studies and canon formations; for Douglas, it exposes the narrowness of a shallow, secular culture steeped in commercial values. Yet neither model considers the effects of pro-sentimentalist positions such as Tompkins's or antisentimentalist positions such as Douglas's on people who are completely left out of the debate. Neither Tompkins's view nor Douglas's view can imagine the course of events that has made the infusion of sentimental rhetoric in AIDS injurious to women's health. The "narrow" parameters of Tompkins and Douglas suggest that in many ways the famous Douglas-Tompkins debate is irrelevant. Sentimental fiction produced and read by white women and liberal Protestant ministers was just one location in which sentimentality materialized. Tompkins and Douglas overlook what Wexler calls "the expansive, imperial project of sentimentalism" (15).

What I am suggesting is that reservations about sentimental rhetoric can be rooted in a variety of conflicting concerns and questions. The interaction of sentimental rhetoric with textual and visual representations of women in AIDS suggests that sentimentality can be reactionary, ultraconservative, and conformist; it is possible to develop a critique of sentimentality that is not inevitably steeped in sexism or misogyny, a view that runs counter to the model that Tompkins and others have erected. The role that sentimental rhetoric plays in conceptions of women in representations of AIDS suggests that sentimental rhetoric should not be exempt from critical scrutiny simply because women's sentimental writing was—and still is—denigrated by masculinized aesthetic politics. Just as we need to be careful that we do not attribute hidden resistance and rebellion to every sentimental representation, we need to be equally careful that we do not deny the presence of conservative impulses in sentimental culture that seemingly promotes a rebellious and resistant stance.[23] The tendency to see sentimentality as utopian resistance to dominant values on the one hand or as an expression of dominant values on the other does not fit the case of women and AIDS, where both patterns exist. Adopting one perspective at the expense of the other can blind interpreters to the ways in which cultural forms validate dominant values even when, in other respects, they are resistant.

Immaculate Infection

This book is organized around the idea of the immaculately infected woman, a Little Eva figure that prevails because of historically ingrained ideas of the biological nature of female sacrifice and caretaking.[24] The image of woman as immaculately infected with HIV—infantilized, asexual, self-denying, and often white—affects all women in different ways, including HIV-negative women of diverse races, ethnicities, and classes.[25] Representations of the "deviant sick" and the "immaculate sick" are interdependent, each of these terms relying on the other for its argument about what women should do and be. To explore representations of the immaculately infected woman, I use Judith Lorber's concept of gender as a social institution, a formal structure similar to language, religion, or the economy (5). As Lorber argues, gender involves a "process of social construction, a system of social stratification, and an institution that structures every aspect of our lives because of its embeddedness in the family, the workplace, and the state, as well as in sexuality, language, and culture" (5). A cultural critique of how women are constructed in representations of AIDS reveals gender as a formidable social institution with accompanying practices and structures that affect every aspect of our lives.

However, in using gender as a central conceptual category, I try to avoid a naive assumption about women and universal sisterhood. For instance, Patty Reagan's statement that "globally, women share a common history of marginality, and now we share a common illness" (153) speaks to the fact that women are HIV infected throughout the world, but the local particularities and histories of that marginality and experience of illness are too heterogeneous for a characterization such as Reagan's. As Nancy A. Hewitt reminds us in "Beyond the Search for Sisterhood," women have historically oppressed other women, and such is the case in representations of women and AIDS.[26] Extending Hewitt's assertion, I explore how more privileged HIV-infected women construct self-representations that maintain not only their own subordination but that of less privileged women—HIV negative as well as positive.

I also draw on the work of various feminist scholars, such as Hazel Carby, who argues in *Reconstructing Womanhood: The Emergence of the Afro-American Woman Novelist* that race is pivotal to ideologies of gender and ideologies of gender are central to constructions of race. Similarly, the work of bell hooks, Patricia Hill Collins, Valerie Smith, Cathy Cohen, and Tamara Jones uses an interlocking lens of race, gender, and sexuality to illuminate the multiple dimensions of identity and oppression. Their perspectives illuminate the ways in which gender and race are intertwined in representations of AIDS. In other words, a gender analysis alone is not going to account for the complex interconnections of racial superiority, gender myths, and illness that structure many of the narratives I investigate. On the other hand, a racial (and class) analysis that fails to acknowledge the social institutions of gender and sexuality will similarly contribute to the belief that AIDS is incidental to women and feminism, thus occluding women's multiple and diverse experiences in the epidemic.

Throughout I focus on how the sentimentalization of women's self-sacrificing care links AIDS and women to a "proper" femininity, and I explore how this rhetorical process coerces women into traditional roles as nursemaids and caretakers. The work of Julia T. Wood and Stephanie

Golden is central to my interpretations of how representations of women's sacrificial caretaking define AIDS narratives. Their scholarship has informed my argument that women's position in the narratives of the epidemic is subsumed by the figure of the good woman, an earnest, didactic role model for a heartless, AIDS-phobic society. One might argue that such a conception of women is harmless given the magnitude of suffering caused by the pandemic. Yet such conceptions create the impression that women themselves are not infected and that their "role" in the pandemic, as well as in society at large, is that of moral guide and caretaker. These visual and print responses make women's complex experiences—most importantly, their experiences as HIV-positive women or women with AIDS—not invisible but secondary and incidental. AIDS becomes an opportunity to rationalize placing women into what Margaret Adams called in a 1971 essay the "compassion trap."[27]

In Chapter 2, "Little Eva Revisited," I examine the famous representation of Little Eva's life and death from tuberculosis in Harriet Beecher Stowe's *Uncle Tom's Cabin* and consider the effect of Stowe's saintly girl character on contemporary representations of women and AIDS. I discuss Little Eva as a paragon of the sacrificial woman and role model for women with AIDS who want to maintain their status as women. I trace Eva's influence in the late Elizabeth Glaser's memoir, *In the Absence of Angels*, and in the speeches of Mary Fisher, a well-connected member of the Republican Party. While I am not chastising these authors for their traditional self-presentations, I do argue that their narratives participate in the social construction of sacrificial, maternal caretaking as women's work alone. Though Little Eva is not the source of this paradigm, she is a good example of its ideology.

Chapter 3, "Absent Mothers and Missing Children," continues an exploration of sacrifice and caretaking in relation to HIV by looking at representations of young children, race, and class. I demonstrate how Perri Klass's novel *Other Women's Children* exposes the racial politics of sentimental deaths of children, both in general and, specifically, in cases of HIV. It is only certain types of children, just as it is only certain types of women, who get to be the suffering, sacrificial Little Eva, the mouthpiece of moral pedagogy and justice. While I analyze Klass's skeptical stance toward Stowe's Little Eva as well as the narrative's complex rewriting of the sentimental novel, I nevertheless point out that *Other Women's Children*, ironically, makes women's position in the epidemic incidental. In other words, the narrative's lack of interest in the mother's complex experiences in the epidemic echoes the legacy of superior Little Eva as the sacrificial mother. This chapter also develops connections between welfare reform and the print and visual representations of women and AIDS by arguing that literature and popular culture operate as extensions of social policy rather than as challenges to social policy. I specifically analyze the similarities between the discourse of welfare and welfare reform and what women are made to represent in AIDS literature. As a counter to the public uses of the good woman pattern, I end the chapter with a discussion of HIV-positive women's experiences as mothers.

Chapter 4, "The Lesbian Mammy," examines the first Hollywood film to address women and AIDS, *Boys on the Side* (1995). Using the interrelated terms of race, gender, and sexuality I investigate what I call the lesbian mammy figure in AIDS discourse, a kind of grown-up, queer version of Stowe's Topsy. *Boys on the Side* portrays an updated Little Eva-like view of American womanhood by constructing HIV in the body of Robin, a white middle-class woman who, when faced with her own mortality, wishes that she had lived a more traditional woman's life. At the time that this film appeared, HIV infection in African American women was skyrocketing, yet the film renders the one African American woman as a caretaking lesbian mammy.

Chapter 5, "What Looks like Progress: Black Feminist Narratives on HIV/AIDS," analyzes three black feminist narratives on HIV/AIDS by black women writers. Each narrative actively undermines the Little Eva/Topsy format; however, only the last novel I discuss, *What Looks like Crazy on an Ordinary Day*, challenges the long-standing identification of sacrificial caretaking as women's work alone. By displacing the caretaking role onto an HIV-negative woman and man, and by making the main character, Ava Johnson, a skeptical voice on the issue, the novel gently questions imposed caretaking and offers instead a model of chosen sacrifice and care.

My conclusion looks briefly at a text that directly confronts the paradigm of women's supposed natural inclination toward sacrificial care. Tiye Milan Selah's short story "An Elegy for Jade" presents black women's creativity and friendship in terms of epidemic illness, family-community history, and loss. "An Elegy for Jade" links medical racism, tuberculosis, and AIDS and portrays an unwavering faith in black women's power and strength, including an outright challenge of the identification of black women with selfless martyrs. It depicts chosen caretaking and sacrifice through the main character who tells the story of her best friend's struggle with HIV.

Through this focus on women's sacrifice and caretaking narratives, it becomes evident that well-meaning responses to AIDS simultaneously resist and reinforce conventional ideas of gender and race. Too often, women's complex experiences are concealed behind an amplified figure of white, sacrificial woman, so that the very discourse that sets itself up as sympathetic deforms the women it is trying to save. AIDS culture teaches us that the use of the "good woman" to "humanize," to make HIV a more permissible topic, is often at all women's expense.

CHAPTER 2

LITTLE EVA REVISITED

> [T]he most ferocious practices in relation to women get
> counted as authentic culture. And women become
> spokespersons for their own dismemberment . . .
>
> Donna Haraway, "A Conversation
> with Donna Haraway"

In times of crisis and great suffering, such as wars and mass epidemics, the figure of the idealized, good woman as modest and selfless, sacrificing her own individuality for the good of family, community, and nation, has repeatedly emerged in Western culture as a balm and source of comfort.[1] This allegorical female figure has also been used to mediate controversial political, social, and moral issues. Slavery in the nineteenth century and the antislavery movement that sprung up in response, and AIDS and AIDS politics in the late twentieth century, are just two examples of national "crisis" and public controversy that have been tempered by evoking white maternal femininity.[2]

For example, Joseph Roach has suggested that the closest analogue to Tony Kushner's world-famous, Pulitzer Prize-winning *Angels in America: A Gay Fantasia on National Themes* is Harriet Beecher Stowe's *Uncle Tom's Cabin* (Savran, 207).[3] Just as Stowe was able to tap into the pulse of the nation and articulate its guilt, sin, and confusion over slavery, so did Kushner transform the stigma of AIDS, homosexuality, and mortality into an entertaining, two-part epic. Both Stowe and Kushner approach their controversial themes through the icon of the devotional mother.[4] Stowe's novel includes a large cast of mothers, many of whom are separated from their children through death or slavery; Kushner populates his work with eccentric yet nurturing angels and surrogate mother figures and caretakers. Each writer presents a radical text that is laced with a conservative nostalgia for feminine nurturance.

However, as suggested in Chapter 1, there are consequences in using the devotional mother icon to make contested topics palatable, even for the good white women who are being idealized. In *Uncle Tom's Cabin*, Stowe's heavy reliance on the image of female self-sacrifice as exemplified by Little Eva means that white superiority and traditional gender roles are nourished at the same time that slavery and male power are exposed and chastised.[5] In AIDS literature, an updated version of the Victorian "angel in the house" contributes to the impression that caretaking is women's "role" in the pandemic. This "angeling" of women also suggests that only women who count as good women, who resemble the self-sacrificing good woman, are fit to teach the nation.

Heterosexual maternal woman operates as a normalizing filter across race and class. In black communities, the victimized woman is used to mediate the stigma of AIDS, suggesting once again a link between public ideologies, policy discourse, and literary strategies.[6] For example, Cathy Cohen argues in *The Boundaries of Blackness: AIDS and the Breakdown of Black Politics* that class and race construct the figure of the heterosexual mother as a "normalizing filter" and moral device. In black communities, the legitimate victims of AIDS are heterosexual mothers and, in particular, their innocent children, who are presented as those most deserving of support and care. Politicians and policy makers use such representations to garner funding and strategically deflect attention away from the moral stigma of black gay men and drug users. In one chapter of her book, Cohen analyzes an NAACP document and comes to the conclusion that "[t]he organization's strategy apparently seeks to circumvent controversial discussions and debates about issues of homosexuality and drug use, allowing instead familiar patriarchal frameworks of innocent children and victimized women to dictate the terms of the debate" (265).[7] Thus, while addressing AIDS and supporting the AIDS movement in the twentieth century are radical literary breakthroughs, presenting the issue through the lens of traditional femininity signals a backlash.

Stowe and Kushner are clearly not the only writers to appreciate the advantages of traditional gender in creating works of art on controversial political themes. Other examples of AIDS literature also employ angel iconography and the good woman as mediator. From the fictional domestic novel *At Risk* by Alice Hoffman, to the sensational nonfiction books *In the Absence of Angels* by Elizabeth Glaser and *Sleep with the Angels: A Mother Challenges AIDS* by Mary Fisher, presenting the heterosexual woman as moral teacher emerges as a strategy for making the taboo issue of AIDS acceptable. Each writer employs traditional domestic values and imagery in presenting her narrative on AIDS.

Hoffman's, Glaser's, and Fisher's writings on AIDS draw on idealized motherhood and white femininity, unwittingly revealing that the ideas of womanhood that we associate with the nineteenth century are alive and well at the turn of the twenty-first century. Just as Stowe used the good mother as a lens through which to address the sexual violence of slavery, these contemporary writers employ the figure of the classic nurturing woman to render "queer" AIDS approachable. Just as Stowe used the figure of Little Eva to present her antislavery and mother-centered argument, these contemporary women writers use a modernized Little Eva as a mechanism for challenging the silences and stigma of AIDS. Yet in so doing, these contemporary writers unwittingly press women into conventional roles of mothers, caretakers, wives.[8]

Little Eva's Cultural Durability: The Legacy of True Womanhood

The figure of Harriet Beecher Stowe's Little Eva, whose innocence, goodness, and Christian death are highlighted in *Uncle Tom's Cabin*, has been a staple of American culture. More than 150 years after her initial appearance, Little Eva, and all that she represents, still structure ideas of American womanhood, race, illness, and compassionate democracy. Proof of Little Eva's legendary cultural power is her own separate entry in *The Oxford Companion to American Literature* and the prominent stand numerous feminist critics take in their skillful defense of her against elitist, masculinist, literary detractors.[9]

Although not one of Little Eva's admirers, Ann Douglas was one of the first to suggest Eva's influence on twentieth-century popular culture. Douglas refers to her as "the predecessor of Miss America, of 'Teen Angel,' of the ubiquitous, everyday, wonderful girl about whom thousands of popular songs and movies have been made" (*Feminization*, 4). Universal

Pictures transferred Little Eva's story to the screen in numerous films, including *Uncle Tom's Cabin* (1927) and *Topsy and Eva* (1927), and core elements of her story repeatedly emerge in contemporary Hollywood films today. Little Eva-like women, whether celebrities like Princess Diana and Mother Teresa or more ordinary women like Mary Fisher and Elizabeth Glaser, blend maternal subjectivity with good woman and good works into a potent symbol of acceptable womanhood.[10] Such ideas can be discerned in films addressing women, domesticity, and death.

The 1998 film *Stepmom* is just one example that features an updated version of Little Eva. *Stepmom* is a story of divorce, suffering children, and a dying mother. An ex-husband, an ex-wife, and the ex-husband's new girlfriend (and wife-to-be) must construct a relationship. The ex-wife, Jackie, exemplifies the ideal, self-sacrificing woman when she puts aside her resentment toward her ex-husband and jealousy toward his much younger fiancée. Jackie does so because she has terminal cancer—a fact she keeps secret throughout most of the film—and she wants to help her rival integrate into the family for the sake of the children.

On the surface, Jackie seems nothing like Little Eva; she's sarcastic, bitter, and worldly whereas Eva is soft-spoken, polite, and ethereal. But as a mother, Jackie is all giving, and it is as a mother that she dies for the sins of her family: the sin of divorce and separation is redeemed through Jackie's death. Like Little Eva, whose "whole being focuses on self-sacrifice" and whom Stowe presents as "the maternal Christ" (Ammons, 164), Jackie is more concerned with preparing her ex-husband's new wife for motherhood than with the cancer in her body.

Jackie does her most important cultural work when she is dying. The closer she is to death, the more fully Jackie embodies the ideal woman; her illness and death are opportunities for her to exemplify selflessness as woman's authentic identity. Like Little Eva, who tells Uncle Tom that she would be glad to die for the slaves—"I *would* die for them, Tom, if I could" (Stowe, 140)—Jackie dies so that her fractured family can be healed. As Little Eva's illness is a spiritual gift to the world, a beacon of light and guidance in time of sin and darkness, Jackie represents the ideal woman who dies in order to support a newly formed heterosexual family.

Jackie, like Little Eva, is more than just another angel too good for this world. Jackie teaches contemporary women how to be good women; she is the ideal American mother-citizen presented to female moviegoers for their edification and example. The pedantic role she assumes is familiar. For example, just before Eva's death, her Aunt Ophelia exclaims, "I wish I were like Eva. She might teach me a lesson" (411). And Topsy, whom Stowe presents as a "heathenish" prankster, is transformed through Eva's love and influence into a black version of the angelic girl. When Eva teaches Ophelia and Topsy, she is implicitly teaching white women readers how to be good women. Then and now, Little Eva models what good women should be and do.

According to Stephanie Golden's study of the paradigm of self-sacrifice in Western culture, women of every racial, ethnic, and class background are encouraged to engage in some form of excessive self-sacrifice (208). Self-denial is a central characteristic of women (Golden, 8, 21, 127, 181). Golden argues that the same sacrificing behavior that would be considered excessive and destructive in men is considered normal behavior in women (75). *Stepmom's* Jackie and Stowe's Little Eva are personifications of good women who are directed away from creating and maintaining a self and identity to focus instead on the development of others. Such a focus releases women from the struggle of having to create a place in a difficult, hostile world; instead, women can form an identity based on other people's developments and redemption. When women behave like Little Eva, "Western culture cheers"; when they don't behave as expected, they are demonized (Golden, 19). It is this excessive ideal of self-sacrifice that links the nineteenth- and twentieth-century images of woman. In the context of AIDS, such a conjunction is deadly.

Little Eva and AIDS Discourse

Contemporary literary and cultural representations of AIDS are populated by the good (innocent children, tender virgins, and vigilant mothers) and the bad ("promiscuous" women and gay men, pathological drug users, "bad" welfare mothers, and contaminated prostitutes). Just as Little Eva imparted stories about gender, race, and acceptable femininity in the age of abolition, her reincarnation today conveys restorative, unsullied white femininity in the age of AIDS. Little Eva revisited saturates the language and culture of AIDS, deflecting attention away from key aspects of women's health—including sexuality and race—and subtly focusing it instead on the preservation of ideal femininity.

Little Eva echoes in the stories of middle-class Kimberly Bergalis, who allegedly contracted HIV through her infected dentist and was presented by both the media and the Bergalis family as an innocent blond virgin. In Bergalis's testimony before a congressional subcommittee, she invoked a dialectic of innocence and guilt when she pleaded, "I've done nothing wrong" (Hood, 158).[11] Just as Little Eva is superior to all the characters in *Uncle Tom's Cabin*, particularly Topsy, Bergalis stands above all the guilty victims of AIDS. Furthermore, in a letter to a friend, Bergalis evokes Little Eva's Christ-like qualities when she writes: "I feel that maybe this illness is the cross I have to carry. . . . Maybe there's something God wants me to do with however much time I have" (Hood, 156). Tellingly, Bergalis's father evokes the trope of Little Eva even more precisely: "I feel she was chosen because she possessed qualities many do not have. . . . [S]ensitive and compassionate . . . she was a very special person who made believers of others. She was chosen for this mission" (Hood, 156).

Kimberly Bergalis's "mission" was not only to carry out the work she and her family began on the Kimberly Bergalis Patient and Provider Protection Act of 1991; her mission, whether she was aware of it or not, was also to serve as a reminder to the nation that white, idealized womanhood prevails, particularly in times of national crisis. Representations of Bergalis conflate infectious illness and homophobia with the ideal woman and thus offer a way to control who counts as a worthy citizen. Unlike Little Eva, Bergalis does not prepare readers for a compassionate response to unpleasant controversy and stigma; Bergalis does not want her audience to sympathize with the traditional outcasts or sufferers of AIDS. In this way, she is a flawed Little Eva, and suggests instead what Linda Singer predicated in *Erotic Welfare: Sexual Theory and Politics in the Age of Epidemic:* that the cultural anxiety and crisis mentality associated with the epidemic would revitalize deeply entrenched fears over sexuality and gender roles. To ward off social breakdown and moral panic, the notion of traditional, infantilized femininity is held up as an antidote (Gorna, 45–71; Kitzinger, 95). The construction of Bergalis as a childlike martyr of the conservative nation-family reinforces the belief that ideal femininity wins out over this epidemic threat to the nation.

Though one aspect of Bergalis's response to being HIV infected was anger, blaming, and vicious homophobia, as Timothy Murphy points out in "The Angry Death of Kimberly Bergalis," an equally significant aspect of her media presentation recalls how her illness gave her life meaning; the meaning that her life came to possess was that of virginal, dying, Christ-like woman. In this way, Bergalis most closely resembles Stowe's Little Eva. The virginal, Christ-like suffering and death connect Bergalis to the True Woman of nineteenth-century America. Mixed in with her blaming and anger is the idealization of the dying woman as a code for traditional gender and racial roles.

Since AIDS is alternately a disregarded, taboo topic and a highly regulated, sensational topic, Little Eva revisited offers a way to mediate the extremes. Eva-like figures break the silence by being the vehicle through which controversial topics are discussed. Their acceptable femininity diffuses the instability and anxiety caused by the open acknowledgment of the taboo topic in the first place. In *Uncle Tom's Cabin,* Stowe uses Eva to speak openly about the brutality of slavery while also offering a model of conservative gender roles and implicit white superiority. Likewise, in much AIDS discourse ideal woman nobly addresses the dishonorable topic of AIDS while also evoking the myth of pure white woman's suffering and death. Modernized Little Eva breaks silence and at the same time stabilizes the instability caused by the breaking of silence. In addition, the respectable, Little Eva-like qualities of Kimberly Bergalis, Murphy argues, allowed people outside of the purported risk groups to question their own risk for AIDS for the first time (84).

Self-sacrificing female subjectivity typified by Stowe's Little Eva and adapted in media accounts reemerges with a vengeance in the controversial AIDS novel *At Risk* by Alice Hoffman, a novel that focuses on AIDS in a child. Although narratives that focus on childhood AIDS may initially treat the child as "abject," they will emphasize his or her prior status—particularly if it is white, middle-class, and suburban—so that the fantasy of American childhood as "pure" can be preserved. Ryan White, the pale, blond-haired hemophiliac who died of AIDS in 1990, can stand for acceptable notions of tragic death because as a hemophiliac he symbolizes acceptable notions of childlike, feminized innocence.

Like Stowe's famous character, Hoffman's ill white girl is presented in terms of domesticity and devoted motherhood. Just as Little Eva served as a model of womanhood for "good" women readers in nineteenth-century America, Hoffman's girl character serves as a model for how women readers should respond to people with AIDS, as well as for how they should behave as women.

Modernizing the Angel in the House

Alice Hoffman's seventh novel, *At Risk,* was inspired by the author's personal fears of losing her young children to AIDS. "When I thought about AIDS," Hoffman writes, "the worst possible thing I could think of was if one of my children had it. That was where my imagination was going" (James, C15). Similar to Stowe, who drew from her experience of losing a child to the Cincinnati plague of 1849 in creating *Uncle Tom's Cabin,* Hoffman uses motherhood and domesticity to win readers' approval of a controversial subject—a rhetorical strategy that contributes to the novel's passion and great feeling, but also to its underlying conservative sensibility. Idealized, white domesticity and self-sacrificing femininity embodied in a girl child mediate the stigma of AIDS.

A gracefully written narrative about a middle-class family torn apart by AIDS, *At Risk* focuses on the Farrells in their idyllic New England suburb north of Boston. Called "Morrow" (rhymes with sorrow and tomorrow, thus forecasting the death to come), the town, with its sandy beaches and former sea captains' houses, attracts tourists and visitors from Boston, especially during the summer. Polly and Ivan Farrell and their two children, eleven-year-old Amanda (who contracted HIV through a blood transfusion while undergoing an emergency appendectomy at six) and eight-year-old Charlie, compose the nuclear family unit around which the narrative is organized. But key characters also include Laurel Smith, a local medium who works with Polly and eventually befriends Amanda, and Brian, a former IV drug user, financially successful pop musician, and gay man with AIDS who works at an AIDS hotline in Boston. A cast of family and friends also contributes to the narrative's plot and development of themes: Polly Farrell's parents, Claire and Al; her work partner, Betsy Stafford; Charlie Farrell's best friend, Sevrin Stafford; Amanda's best friend, Jessie Eagan; her gymnastics coach, Jack Eagan; and her pediatrician, the Harvard-educated Dr. Ed Reardon.

Polly Farrell is a full-time, stay-at-home mother and a freelance photographer who uses whatever money she makes from her work to supplement the family's income. When the novel opens, she is professionally engaged in what her two children sarcastically call the "Casper Project" since it involves the photographing of seances conducted by Laurel Smith. Ivan Farrell, Polly's husband, is an astronomer and university professor who is very proud of his son, Charlie, a budding scientist obsessed with prehistoric creatures. Amanda, who exhibits dramatic symptoms of AIDS by the end of the first chapter, wants to become a professional gymnast; she is very determined and talented.

The plot tracks Amanda's decline, from the first vague fevers that lead to a series of blood tests and biopsies, to a diagnosis of AIDS, subsequent hospitalizations, and finally, Amanda on her deathbed dictating her makeshift last will and testament. Other central elements include the emotional and social toll AIDS takes on each member of the Farrell family, in particular, the cruel prejudice, social rejection, and isolation the Farrells experience owing to their friends' and fellow townspeople's ignorance of AIDS transmission. Each character grapples with fears of mortality, which find voice in intense and disturbing dreams and daytime reveries, and the shunning incidents mount with each new chapter.

Polly Farrell's friends and neighbors are distant, and they purposely fail to inquire about Amanda when they meet Polly in the market or gas station. Charlie Farrell loses his best friend Sevrin because the boy's mother will not allow him to play with Charlie for fear of contamination. At school, Charlie's classmates refuse to sit next to him, and Amanda's ridicule her. Polly and Ivan, together with the doctor, Ed Reardon, have to fight school officials and parents' groups to allow Amanda to stay in school. It is not just physical death encroaching on this family, but a social death.

The ignorance and fear of the people of Morrow send each family member into isolation or a search for comfort from an outside source. Friendless Charlie goes to his pond to collect specimens and ruminate about science and prehistoric creatures. Amanda retreats to her room where she listens to Madonna and bravely tries to perform her gymnastics routine. Polly fantasizes about an affair with Ed Reardon. After Amanda's diagnosis, Polly spends a lot of time talking with Amanda's physician; the two adults experience a mutual attraction but limit the expression of their feelings to one passionate kiss. Sensing Polly's emotional withdrawal and suffering deeply from the shock of Amanda's diagnosis, Ivan Farrell can't concentrate on the scientific paper he is scheduled to deliver at a conference in Florida; instead, he spends his time calling Brian, whose knowledge and sensitivity shepherd Ivan through the pain and bewilderment of his daughter's terminal illness. Amanda, though she thinks about her death, bravely pursues her dream of becoming a gymnast despite bodily pain.

Hoffman skillfully uses domestic values and a realistic writing style to show how a financially secure family with "average" problems—Ivan is a distracted workaholic, Amanda and Charlie are sibling rivals—is "at risk." As a result, the novel challenges the us/them paradigm that characterized AIDS discourse in the 1980s by arguing that anyone, even the "least likely," such as Amanda Farrell, can contract HIV. Hoffman explains, "I wanted the novel to be about somebody who would seem like an All-American girl, the least likely person to get it, in the least likely place" (James, C15). It is precisely this "All-American girl" sensibility that brings to mind Stowe's Little Eva and the ideology of female self-sacrifice.

At first glance, it may seem strange to compare Alice Hoffman's Amanda Farrell to Harriet Beecher Stowe's Little Eva. Little Eva appears in a famous mid-nineteenth-century antislavery narrative, and Amanda Farrell emerges in a late-twentieth-century novel about an infectious epidemic associated with illicit sexuality and criminal drug use. In addition Stowe's dying girl character's Christianity organizes her worldview and every aspect of her personality. At Risk substitutes athleticism for Christianity, making the narrative seem more a novelization of A. E. Housman's "To an Athlete Dying Young" than a reworking of Little Eva. The two girl characters have blond hair and die, but this seems to be their only similarity.

But, in fact, At Risk modernizes the Little Eva figure by replacing her with a more secular, physical girl character. Amanda does not believe she is in contact with heaven the way that Little Eva does, and the reader repeatedly sees Amanda as a character with worldly ambitions, unlike Little Eva. By page 3 of the novel, however, Amanda is exhibiting subtle symptoms of AIDS, and the language of the text begins to spiritualize her illness, just as Stowe spiritualizes Eva's tuberculosis.[12] Amanda's etherealized body signals her association with the nineteenth-century concept of the cult of true womanhood.[13] Just as Eva is "no more contained in one place than a sunbeam or a summer breeze" (Stowe, 230), Amanda is "one made up not of flesh but of points of brilliant light" (Hoffman, 9), so "weightless, you'd think she was flying straight into the sun" (188–89). Disembodying Amanda Farrell links her to a literary tradition of white, ethereal femininity and innocence and turns her into a lens through which controversial subjects can be addressed.

Stowe's novel uses Little Eva to convince its white readers that black families under slavery deserve the same Christian charity as white families. Hoffman uses the death of a white middle-class girl and the suffering endured by her family to attack the prejudice and intolerance aimed at more traditional outcasts with AIDS. The entire Farrell family becomes the vehicle of compassion for the more unacceptable people with AIDS. In other words, as white readers of *Uncle Tom's Cabin* are asked to transfer their feelings of sympathy for Little Eva to the enslaved, black Uncle Tom, heterosexual readers of *At Risk* are being asked to transfer their sympathy and identification with Hoffman's dying girl character and her devastated family to gay men and drug users with AIDS. As Catharine O'Connell puts it in an essay on Stowe, mainstream white readers can "feel the suffering of an/Other only when the Other has become them" (34). Like Stowe, who stresses similarity between Little Eva and Uncle Tom, Hoffman subtly plays up similarities between Amanda Farrell, the young girl dying of AIDS, and Brian, the gay man and former drug user with AIDS, by describing both characters in transcendent, otherworldly language. In a sense, Brian becomes the "queer" white version of Uncle Tom.

The transcendent language used to spiritualize Amanda's body in order to infuse her illness and death with meaning is also used to describe Brian's ill body. In one scene, Ivan talks about the kind of children's literature he reads to Amanda and Charlie, literature in which mythological heroes are "plucked from death and set into the sky" so that "flesh and blood is transformed into blinding light" (172). Shortly thereafter, Brian's body—his queer white flesh and blood—is described as "dissolving": "Brian is barely here, he is already looking at something far away, something in another dimension no one else can see" (173). Queer Brian and good Amanda are linked through the rhetorical strategy of describing them in spiritual, disembodied terms.

Both Little Eva and Amanda induce feelings of sympathy and transfer them to social outcasts (Brian) and the "lowly" (Uncle Tom), because the two girls stand out as exceptional role models; even though they are children, each symbolizes womanly self-sacrifice and the mother-citizen. Little Eva stands out because of her precocious spirituality and faith in God, and the more ill she becomes the more "womanly" she seems. Her father notes that there is "a touching and womanly thoughtfulness about her now, that everyone noticed" (385). Amanda stands out because of her single-minded pursuit of gymnastics, and she is described by her mother as "the only one with any real purpose" (8). Like Eva, Amanda also approaches death with a precocious acceptance.

Amanda prepares her mother and her best friend for her death by withdrawing from them so that they will get used to being without her: "She's already started spending less time with her mother. Now it's time to do the same with Jessie" (187). Although Amanda is afraid of death, she is in less denial than her mother and friend; her preparation suggests her singularity and exemplar status (188, 270). The medium Laurel Smith, an adult version of Amanda, is more comfortable with death, the afterlife, and the supernatural. Laurel wins Amanda's trust and Amanda confides in her. In contrast to Amanda's bigoted schoolmates and neighbors, Laurel seeks Amanda out and feels at ease with her illness and approaching death; she guides Amanda to the next world. It is Laurel, not Polly, to whom Amanda discloses her fear of death, her wish not to upset her mother (which is why the girl withdraws from her), and her greatest wish: to have her braces removed (226, 243). Their sudden and intense relationship, combined with their similar physical and personality features, suggests the kind of woman Amanda would have been—one a lot like Laurel Smith.[14]

Similarities between Stowe and Hoffman are not limited to their dying heroines. Like Stowe's novel, Hoffman's narrative suggests that women's culture is preferable to the rational, scientific culture of men. Hoffman explores how AIDS threatens science's authority. At one point, Ivan "can no longer think the way he must to do his work at the institute; questions no longer have answers" (184). Amanda's doctor "feels like a charlatan" (250). Charlie "really believed that, given enough time, science could answer any question, but it cannot" (83). Pondering the stars and prehistoric life remain viable for Ivan and his alter ego, Charlie, only because they represent creativity and mystery. "[P]ure science" as the privileged domain with exact answers is exposed as vulnerable and useless before the power of mortality and "the random path of a virus" (56).

The threat to the family in *Uncle Tom's Cabin* is slavery, a system created by rampant male greed and capitalist individualism,[15] while the threat to the family in *At Risk* is AIDS, a natural disaster symbolized by a wasp in the kitchen in the novel's opening scene. Perhaps the most dramatic foreshadowing of the domestic anguish to follow, the wasp functions as a metaphor for AIDS: "There is a wasp in the kitchen. Drawn by the smell of apricot jam, lazy from the morning's heat, the wasp hovers above the children" (3). A force of nature, the wasp is a potent, "pregnant" energy that "hovers above the children" and threatens the Farrells' love and cohesiveness. Significantly, Ivan and his son, Charlie, respond to the wasp with scientific fascination, while Polly and Amanda, sensing danger and threat, want it dead. Here, the separate spheres of male rationality couched in science and female intuitiveness and emotionality emerge. Amanda's and Charlie's responses encapsulate the two realms: "Get it out of here!" says Amanda; "No way!" says Charlie (3). Just as Stowe's famous novel attacks slavery while subtly reproducing white superiority and conservative gender roles, Hoffman's novel attacks AIDS discrimination while promoting a revitalization of white Victorian gender ideology and systemic heterosexism.

Critical Responses to *At Risk*

Most critical reactions to Alice Hoffman's novel ignore the implications for women of an idealized girl character with AIDS. When Hoffman's novel was presented in 1988 at the American Booksellers Association conference under glitzy lights and with a glossy cover, best-selling gay novelist David Leavitt quickly discerned that the book's favorable public reception was linked to homophobia and the politics of the innocent victim. Leavitt pointed to the fact that *Newsweek* had given a mixed review to Paul Monette's memoir *Borrowed Time* while praising Hoffman's *At Risk* for its heartfelt, family qualities. Leavitt and other commentators have argued that Hoffman's seemingly liberal, humanistic novel is "set against" gay men and other social outcasts associated with AIDS (Nelson, 170).

James Morrison maintains that the "sympathy elicited for the 'innocent' derives precisely from the encodement of *that which they are not*—a figure, that is, of insidious otherness" (quoted in Nelson, 170).[16] Amanda Farrell's characterization suggests that she is explicitly *not* one of "the already stigmatized" or one of the already "most vulnerable victims" of AIDS.[17] She, like Little Eva, is an "insider," loved by everyone, and this aspect of her character is consistently emphasized in the novel. In fact, Amanda's favorable identity *prior* to AIDS is crucial to the fictional expression of her life after she is diagnosed. The narrative also includes language that undermines Hoffman's stated theme that everyone with the virus is innocent. According to Ivan Farrell, Amanda has "been murdered" and "if he ever could find out who donated the blood Amanda got, he would break that person's neck, he would listen to the bones snap" (65). Though Dr. Judith Shapiro, Amanda's Boston AIDS specialist, reminds Ivan that "no one is at fault" (mouthing one of Hoffman's themes), the language here constructs Amanda as the victim of the absent, hideous blood donor who looms throughout the story and serves as a foil to Amanda (69).

Controversy over *At Risk* has also added to a larger debate over the ways in which the realities of characters with HIV infection and AIDS are overshadowed by the fearful responses and denial of those characters who do not test positive. For example, one of the earliest television movies to address AIDS, *An Early Frost*, charts the reactions of a white heterosexual mother and father and their neighbors to a gay character with AIDS. The gay man and his male partner function as vehicles for the other characters'—and, implicitly the viewers'—cathartic release. Joseph Cady's "Teaching about AIDS through Literature in a Medical School Curriculum" discusses *At Risk* as an example of this evasiveness by noting "how tenacious and subtle the cultural avoidance" of AIDS is in Hoffman's novel (239). While some read *At Risk* as a humane expression of Alice Hoffman's "compassion for every AIDS victim regardless of how he or she contracted the virus," as Judith Laurence Pastore proposes (40), others interpret the narrative as one more example of heterosexism.[18]

But the question I have been raising is not so much whether Hoffman's novel approaches AIDS from the standpoint of the gay person with AIDS or the heterosexual onlooker, but how AIDS becomes an opportunity to revamp deeply conservative conceptions of gender. There is no doubt that the devotional mother/good woman icon is exploited to de-gay AIDS, and that such a strategy epitomizes widespread homophobia and racism, but there are serious consequences of such a process for ideas about women, whatever their sexual identity. *At Risk*, like many print and visual responses to AIDS, subtly reworks views grounded in the nineteenth-century figure of the suffering, sacrificial woman. Idealized femininity as "device" reiterates the stereotype that women's main purpose in life is to sacrifice for others, and that women's most important role—even when they are HIV positive—is as childlike moral teachers and compassionate educators. It is this insight that is often overlooked in much writing on the novel.

Whether critics admire or detest Hoffman's narrative, whether they see it as transgressive or as conservative, the female child dying of AIDS in the novel is also set against women; the presentation of AIDS in an "innocent" girl reinforces the notion that HIV-infected women are either desexed innocent victims or deviant cesspools of infection. In relying so heavily on the Little Eva prototype, Hoffman's narrative unwittingly glamorizes the very gender roles that intensify women's (and girls') risk and otherness. So while it is crucial to explore the cultural politics of portraying a young girl with AIDS in juxtaposition with gay male sexuality, health, and cultures, it is equally important to consider how a female-coded infantilized innocence affects women's sexualities, cultures, and health.[19]

For the Sake of Gender

Narratives of Little Eva recur in countless contemporary representations of women with AIDS whose stories are judged to be "the saddest stories" (Kitzinger, 98). Her legacy continually animates, not only contemporary fiction on AIDS, but the testimonies, speeches, and media images of adult, HIV-positive women. Even though these women are infected, they can still be thought of as "saviors of the nation." While there are numerous examples of women who refuse standard ideas of AIDS and of traditional gender roles, in particular, the role of the good woman,[20] many famous—and ordinary—women evoke the "good mother, "the ministering angel," "the injured innocent victim," the one who really doesn't *deserve* AIDS, as a strategy of self-protection against stigma and social rejection. The most effective of these constructions is that of the maternal woman as selfless nurturer.

Little Eva's legacy emerges in twentieth-century women's memoirs and speeches, in which the maternalizing and spiritualizing conceptions of women frame the autobiographical stories. Here benevolent womanhood prevails. A reoccurring theme in these memoirs is that HIV infection for women threatens their very identity as "women"—unless women can evoke Little Eva—and at the same time offers women the opportunity to symbolize the ultimate in American womanhood.[21]

Well-known representations of two famous women with AIDS, Elizabeth Glaser and Mary Fisher, recall Stowe's strategy of approaching controversial issues through the lens of maternal self-abnegation. Each woman's published narrative conveys and creates a married heterosexual woman's and mother's perspective on AIDS intertwined with a more subtle narrative of the self-sacrificing woman as symbolic solution to AIDS.

Elizabeth Glaser, devoted Hollywood wife of the former TV star Paul Michael Glaser, spoke of her life as a woman with AIDS at the 1992 Democratic convention, and HIV-positive Mary Fisher, dubbed "the Christmas angel" by journalist Maureen Dowd, spoke at the 1992 Republican convention.[22] When Glaser died of AIDS in December 1994, *People* magazine placed her photograph on its cover, and writer David Ellis compiled a list of tributes from friends and celebrities under the heading "Remembering an Angel of Hope." Glaser was called a "camp counselor," a "mother bear," and "just a mother who happened to have two children with AIDS" (46–53). Her own experiences as an adult woman with AIDS were overshadowed by the image of devoted mother who launched the first Pediatric AIDS Fund after the death of her young daughter. Glaser's 1991 autobiography, *In the Absence of Angels: A Hollywood Family's Courageous Story*, similarly focuses on her maternal activism.

As we read Glaser's autobiography, the profile of the ideal woman emerges. She frames her identity in terms of how she addresses her children's and her husband's needs.[23] About her sexuality, Glaser writes that she was a young woman of "prom girl innocence" from an upper-middle-class family (42). In telling her story, she subtly reinforces a key feature of AIDS: the division between gay white male communities and the general (heterosexual) population, as well as between "good," monogamous, married women and "bad," sexually active, "single" women:

> They explained that there had been a lot of infected blood at Cedars-Sinai
> Hospital in the early years of the epidemic because it is located on the edge

of West Hollywood, which is predominantly gay. They asked me if I had ever had any sexual relationships with anyone other than Paul. I laughed because the question seemed so stupid. I hadn't even kissed anyone else except my husband since the day I met him. (47–48)

Glaser conceptualizes AIDS as a disease originating with white gay men who dwell on "the edge"; her remarks also hint at the degree to which she has internalized good woman as faithful, quiet, and devoted. Though she attended college in the sixties, she refers to the era of antiwar protests and other social movements as a time when "buildings were being blown up" and when she lost her "innocence" (42). Glaser reproduces traditional gender roles in her marriage as well. She writes that she and her housekeeper "were always trying to find new ways to keep the baby quiet when Paul was working at home" (28) and that "women talk about their babies the way men talk about sports" (29).

Glaser's activism emerges when she and her daughter test positive; her goal becomes making children's experiences in the epidemic visible, a crucial, important goal which she achieved. However, she frames her activism in terms of saving her children, not in terms of her own or other women's health.[24] She laces her narrative with the imagery of the good mother and feminine sacrifice. For example, while Paul Glaser kept a grueling work schedule, his wife was left to deal with the health crisis on her own: "Paul was working night and day. It was as if Ari and I were on an island" (38). Although not happy about coping alone, Glaser concludes that "it's a duty I never once considered shirking" (49). About her own health, she says: "As far as my own physical condition was concerned, I knew I had to stay strong so I could save my children" (49).

But her story includes an increasingly radical awareness of power: "When I have met with people in power it's usually because they think I am one of them. In terms of color and economics, yes, I look the same, but I don't feel I have much in common with them. My goals are not their goals. They want to protect what is theirs. They want a kinder and gentler America for them, but not necessarily for others" (177). The more Glaser fights on behalf of children, including her own, the more she moves out of her traditional role of mother into the world of fund-raising and Washington politics: "I was much more of a victim when I was just taking care of my family, trying to keep our lives normal without taking any risks. Becoming active in the fight against AIDS made me realize I'm not a victim. I have power and I can work for change" (177). As a result of these experiences, she develops a critique of power as well as strategies for getting what she wants, and she also becomes aware, perhaps for the first time, of her racial and economic privilege.

HIV-positive Mary Fisher, called "the world's most famous mommy with AIDS," creates a self-representation that is even more explicitly evocative of Little Eva (Dowd, 33, 34). Fisher intersperses family pictures throughout her published collection of speeches, *Sleep with the Angels: A Mother Challenges AIDS*.[25] Family photos in the book include numerous shots of her two young sons involved in various physical activities: wading in the ocean, running along the shoreline of white sandy beaches, or playing baseball with their infected mother (Fisher's children are HIV negative). Also prevalent are shots of Fisher holding the youngest son in her arms while the older son watches. As Torie Osborne observes, Fisher brings a "feminine force, a maternal fierceness, into AIDS" (Dowd, 35).

Fisher describes herself as a mother, a "longtime Republican," and a pilgrim "on the road to AIDS." Similar to Stowe's and Hoffman's use of ominous foreshadowing is Fisher's repeated evocation of her inevitable death and the fate of her orphaned sons.[26] She emphasizes her identity as a dead mother just as Stowe and Hoffman repeatedly forecast the inevitable deaths of their angelic girl characters. Nowhere is Fisher's mixture of maternal vigilance and fixation on death more apparent than in the opening chapter of *Sleep with the Angels*, significantly titled "A Letter to My Children":

> Tonight when I tucked each of you into bed, I said to you what you've heard me say every night of your lives. Since the moment you came from my body, Max, and the hour you were placed in my arms, Zachary, I have known that I would, one day, need to give you up.
>
> And so, each night, I rehearse for the day when I must give you over. That is why as I reach for the day's last kiss and hug, you always hear me say the same four words, "Sleep with the angels." (23)

The passage blends the maternal, the sacred, and the domestic into a potent image reminiscent of nineteenth-century motherhood used today in the service of AIDS education. Here, it is her death, not the child's, that is evoked, but the image is one of separation of mother and child. Even religious conservatives who believe that AIDS is a punishment might soften after reading this passage about her soon-to-be-motherless sons. (Whether religious conservatives would be able to transfer their sympathy from Fisher and her boys to gay men, sex workers, and injection drug users is questionable.) As if sensing the political implications of her own words, Fisher goes on to explain that she's "more mother than crusader," but her text reveals how the role of mother is far from politically neutral. The American tendency to use the narrative of mother-child separation to frame social problems creates more than tears; it creates social policies (Cvetkovich, 127). Fisher's example illustrates that even in a woman's most painful and seemingly private experiences, conventional ideas of women emerge and become the unspoken solution. The cultural stereotype of conventional motherhood superimposed on the story of AIDS shapes the way that Fisher presents herself.

By the end of 1992, awareness about women and AIDS was exploding in the popular media and in HIV/AIDS communities. Many activists, led by women who had formerly been feminist and lesbian health educators, were fighting with the Centers for Disease Control over its male-centered definition of AIDS. As many reporters, health care professionals, academics, and activists asserted, the official definition of AIDS meant that women were dying of AIDS without having received an AIDS diagnosis. The risk of AIDS to women, according to Elinor Burkett, was "underestimated and underpublicized. Most ominously, it meant that gynecologists weren't warned to consider persistent problems as possible signs of HIV infection, consigning women to late diagnoses and early deaths" (Burkett, 194). Burkett further explained that "the average white gay man with HIV lives 39 months after his diagnosis with full-blown AIDS; the average woman survives 27.4 weeks after her diagnosis. HIV-infected women are one-third more likely to die without an AIDS-defining condition than are HIV-infected men" (192).

However, Fisher's response to these statistics on women and AIDS recalls Marilyn Quayle's suggestion offered at the 1992 Republican National Convention: women should return to "their essential natures." In one speech, Fisher describes women's central activity in the epidemic as "wrapping the family in the quilt" (*Sleep*, 57). In a brilliant political ploy to reframe AIDS as a "family issue," thus appropriating the family values rhetoric of the conservative right, Fisher replaces the phrase "AIDS communities" with her newly created term "the American HIV/AIDS family." However, she also politely questions the assertion that women have been "invisible." Fisher asks gay men to "teach us, especially as women, to unite with all who will support us—lest for the sake of gender we weaken the family whose only strength is found in unity" (54). In other words, the unity and cohesiveness of the newly constituted HIV/AIDS family is more important than raising questions about women's rights, women's medical experiences, or women's needs. To raise such issues is to risk seeming divisive and mean.

Fisher argues that "our role—*my* role—in this family is not first to lead, but to serve" (*Sleep*, 56). Here Fisher uses the rhetoric of the traditional heterosexual family and the separate spheres—men lead, women serve—to render the queer AIDS family acceptable. In her speech, controversy over women's access to treatment and research becomes a metaphor for women's place as symbolized by the AIDS Quilt.[27] Disputes over women's inclusion are irrelevant since women have been given their emblematic "place" in the HIV/AIDS family:

> The place of women in American history has not always been recognized. But yesterday morning I stood on the platform preparing to read names, waiting for the Quilt to be unfurled, knowing that the history of American women would be rolled out before me.
>
> Because, more than a century ago, before radios and telephones and fax machines; before Dorothea Dix humanized mental health and *Uncle Tom's Cabin* shook the morality from slavery; before many American women had learned to read, there was the quilting bee, the weekly community of women. . . . When, a century later, some San Francisco friends decided that each name of lost loved ones should be captured on a Quilt, the history of women was woven into the history of AIDS in America.
>
> Therefore, we women need not fight to find our place. It has been given to us. We need only be true to who we are, women; to do what women have done through the centuries: Wrap the family in the Quilt. (56–57)

By linking American women's relationship to HIV to their historical roles as quilters and moral teachers, Fisher enacts a political strategy that many women of diverse racial and class backgrounds have used brilliantly in this country. But Fisher, like Stowe and many other writers who evoke women's special culture, does not consider the material consequences of such a strategy. Instead of empowering women to see themselves as complete, complex people, women are being told to keep the AIDS family together, even if doing so means to downplay or minimize their own mental and physical health. Putting the needs of family and community before their own needs is a fundamental feature of women's socialization in Western culture, and often a basic barrier to their accessing health care and treatment; yet Fisher suggests this is the "solution."

Although Fisher acknowledges the darker aspects of the epidemic, for example, prejudice and intolerance, she, like the sentimental heroine, offers herself as an example and solution. Rather than engaging in collective social protest, she encourages women to assume their traditional roles. Although she briefly mentions that she felt anger toward her deceased husband for infecting her with HIV, in general she avoids complex feelings such as anger and rage, feelings she has kept at bay for "the sake of the children."[28]

Almost every one of Fisher's speeches epitomizes this nostalgic view of women as forgiving, selfless martyrs, even when infected by men who may have known they were HIV positive and engaged in unprotected sex anyway—which is, in fact, a common occurrence. Just as Stowe emphasizes Little Eva's brave resignation to death and Hoffman repeatedly describes Amanda as too good for this world, Fisher extols the idealized construction of woman as one who sacrifices herself in order to dispense spiritual lessons to readers and fellow Americans. A gendered aspect influences this particular effort to "soften" the grim reality of living with HIV/AIDS: woman as self-abnegating saint.

In Fisher's next book of speeches, *I'll Not Go Quietly: Mary Fisher Speaks Out*, which was published two years after *Sleep with the Angels*, she has clearly begun to think more deeply about the politics of women and AIDS and has revised her view of women's place: "It occurred to me that perhaps one thing I could do is be more bold in speaking as a woman to other women" (*Quietly*, 107). In this book, Fisher again self-presents as the devoted mother, interposing pictures of her young sons at play, in the ocean, and in the family's built-in swimming pool;

she continues to evoke her death by repeatedly asking her audiences to think of her motherless sons in the near future. Nevertheless, *I'll Not Go Quietly* possesses a subtle feminist edge that is absent in her first book.

In one speech addressed to doctors and health-care workers, Fisher says, "We know less today about the course of HIV in women than in men because research has been influenced by prejudice and politics" (*Quietly*, 139). Her speech includes the following scenario derived from her communication with numerous women:

> I cannot count the number of times I've been told variations of the following story. An ordinary woman—you, me, your wife, one of our friends— goes to an ordinary physician. The woman is in her twenties or thirties or forties. . . . Having reviewed her life and having scanned the HIV statistics in America, she says to her physician, "Perhaps I could have a test for AIDS." And she hears the response, "You don't need that—you're not that kind of woman." (*Quietly*, 135)

Here the good woman/bad woman paradigm structuring these kinds of responses prevents women from taking care of their bodies and lives. But more important, the passage unwittingly exposes how historically entrenched ideas about women shape the health care delivery system.

With this view, Fisher moves into new territory and begins to criticize the ways in which women with AIDS are represented and treated, thus revealing gender roles as an unacknowledged barrier and as an ideological response to the panic created by AIDS:

> I was raised to think of the ideal woman as someone of great virtue. To be feminine is to be desirable. And society tells me that AIDS is repulsive. . . . I do ask that, in your practice and in your healing, you recognize that women who are, or who may be, HIV-positive are still women.
>
> We may define our life worth according to some distant sense of virtue and morality, taught to us by a parish priest or *Father Knows Best* or an alcoholic mother. It does not matter how we learned it. What matters is that, if we come to you believing that to be HIV-positive is to be without virtue, part of your healing must be aimed there, at the belief that we are not worthy. (*Quietly*, 136–37)

The ideology of femininity and the institutions that reproduce gender through cultural, religious, intellectual, and familial categories are alluded to through Fisher's inclusion of the 1950s popular television series *Father Knows Best*. Her plea for understanding from doctors signals her awareness of the impact of normative femininity, with which many women grapple when they test positive. The problem for most HIV-positive women is that they no longer possess the qualities that count as "woman"—one who is clean and virtuous—in light of having a disease that renders them "not woman." They must therefore perform idealized femininity, become immaculately infected women, as a way to camouflage their infected status.

However, Fisher soon retreats from social critique and embraces essentialist views of women, even as she vigorously includes women's issues in her "campaign for compassion" speeches. In the following passage, she implores physicians to encourage HIV-positive women to keep their roles as mothers and lovers:

> If it is a uniquely feminine experience to have a child nursing at one's breast—and I can assure you that it is—there is also something uniquely feminine that HIV-positive women can bring to their roles as caregivers. (*Quietly*, 137, 138)

Women's reproductive capacity is transformed into myths and fantasies of women's essential nature. What is most astounding about this passage is that numerous women with HIV have said that while women's traditional role as caregiver is extremely important to women and cultures, the unexamined expectation that women should care is also what puts them at risk for contracting HIV and for neglecting their health once they test positive or become ill (Burkett; Corea; Rudd and Taylor; Wood). Fisher's suggestion that doctors advise women to maintain their caregiving roles also seems naive, since for most women caregiving is hardly a role they can assume one day and then abandon for something else the next.

As with Little Eva and Amanda Farrell, Fisher's illness makes her a "more angel than ordinary" woman, although she insists that there is nothing unique about her and that she should not be seen as a "hero." In her speech "Make Me No Hero," she begins to wonder about her fame: "I was no longer sure that inviting people to 'look at me' was such a good idea. . . . It was, I thought, the right time to explain that I am not a hero"

(*Sleep*, 111–12). At the same time, however, she continually divulges that she's not gay, she's not an IV-drug user, she's not a hemophiliac, she's not poor, and that she "became infected in marriage" (*Sleep*, 28, 49). As the role model for mothers with AIDS, an image that emerges in her numerous television appearances, speeches, and books, Fisher unknowingly presents sentimental gender roles as a viable response to AIDS.[29] An underlying subtext of her speeches is that an HIV-positive woman who still wants to be considered "good woman" should frame herself as a devoted, vigilant, selfless mother; if she does not have children or if her race, class, and/or sexual identification complicate her ability to assume the guise of the good mother, she must repress those parts of her identity that are in conflict with this myth and exaggerate any aspect of her identity that fits.

It is not that Fisher's self-presentation indicates a flaw in her personality or political values; rather, her speeches suggest both the effect of AIDS on ideas about women and the effects of conventional ideas about women on representations of AIDS. Fisher's and Glaser's writings indicate how the power of gender ideology emerges. They show that the actual material realities of any woman's life are often less important than how her life situation can be abstracted into symbols of morality for public consumption and gender management.

While Elizabeth Glaser's writing conveys a more activist sensibility, both she and Fisher seem unconcerned with the impact of gender on their bodies and self-presentations. The pervasiveness of the good woman conception in AIDS print and visual culture suggests that our society is constantly transforming women into icons. Such a practice is larger than any individual woman's—beginning with Stowe's—gender and racial politics. In the next chapter, I pursue the theme of race and gender in literary and visual conceptions of AIDS in terms of another popular figure—the innocent baby.

ABSENT MOTHERS AND MISSING CHILDREN

> Dying children are the sweet creamy centers of
> literature.
>
> Perri Klass, *Other Women's Children*

> The devaluation of mother is always at once the
> devaluation of women.
>
> Andrea Liss, "The Body in Question: Rethinking
> Motherhood, Alterity, and Desire"

Representations of children in AIDS discourse are often cited as evidence of the "changing face of AIDS," but images of dying babies also embody moral ideas about who deserves AIDS and who does not.[1] Appeals and policies made on behalf of ill children are also coded attempts to preserve and control cultural ideas about childhood, motherhood, citizenship, and the nation. The child figure is simultaneously a way to convey and create conceptions of race and innocence and produce conceptions of women as good (or bad) mothers. While dead children and babies speak to the historical fact of childhood mortality in the epidemic, their deaths offer opportunities to reassert what counts as childhood and motherhood in the United States. Such symbolic uses of children's deaths in representations of AIDS come with consequences for both women and children.

Select images of ill children divert attention away from the actual everyday realities of children and women with HIV and AIDS. Not only are the lived complexities of most children concealed behind the spectacle of the dying (often white) child, so are the lived complexities of most women. Furthermore, as discussed in Chapter 2, just as only certain types of women get to be the suffering, sacrificial Little Eva, the mouthpiece of moral pedagogy and compassionate democracy, only certain children get to symbolize childhood AIDS. The effects of the dying child on cultural understandings of children and women are neither new nor unique to narratives on AIDS. Once again, the legacy of *Uncle Tom's Cabin* emerges as a central paradigm in maintaining traditional ideas of race, childhood, and motherhood in the context of a national epidemic.

This chapter explores contemporary narratives on babies, HIV, and motherhood as imagined in fiction and film and argues that literature and popular culture often function as extensions of social policy, even when these same cultural forms are purportedly providing a humane perspective on HIV/AIDS. One contemporary novel, *Other Women's Children*, exposes the racial politics of sentimental deaths of children in literature, both in general and, specifically, in terms of HIV. While I genuinely celebrate *Other Women's Children*'s skeptical stance toward Stowe's Little Eva as well as its complex rewriting of the sentimental novel, Klass ironically makes women's position in the epidemic incidental and contributes to dubious symbolic uses of women in the epidemic. The narrative's stunning lack of interest in the mother's complex experiences in the epidemic dovetails with the traditional paradigm that created the idealized, superior Little Eva in the first place.

The made-for-television film *A Place for Annie*, a narrative that constructs HIV-positive women as infectious threats to their children, suggests some of the consequences of this subsumption of the mother's experience under that of the child. Comparing this view of women in the film to similar representations of women and HIV infection in popular medical discourse shows that medical discourse and television "mutually feed upon each other."[2]

The voices of women with HIV and / or struggling with poverty are curiously absent from public debate. Both the discourse of AIDS and welfare reform turn on the implicit idealization of white-middle class motherhood as model and ideal, suggesting, once again, that controlling the categories of good woman and childhood is more urgent than providing food and health care for single mothers and their children. By using the words and actions of HIV-positive mothers as a paradigm, we will neither conflate women with their children by rendering mothers as self-effacing angels or selfish devils, nor ignore the realities of women and children with HIV infection and AIDS.

AIDS and the Cultural Ideal of Childhood

Jenny Kitzinger's research into the social construction of childhood in campaigns to prevent child sexual abuse sheds light on how ideas about childhood are used in AIDS discourses. Kitzinger argues that child sexual abuse campaigns, while well-meaning and ostensibly organized and administered to protect and educate children, unwittingly exacerbate children's powerlessness and risk. Power is rarely addressed because an unacknowledged goal of child abuse prevention campaigns is the preservation of traditional power, which relies upon the production of an uncomplicated, decontextualized, nostalgic view of childhood. As a result, children are typically represented without context, agency, or personality; instead, they are either innocent victims or lying minxes, a moral opposition of good and bad also commonly found in narratives on AIDS. Campaigns against childhood sexual abuse should be supported, no matter how contradictory or flawed, just as narratives of children with AIDS should be disseminated, no matter how rooted in traditional hierarchies of race and gender. But representations of children in either context are neither neutral nor beyond cultural critique. In the context of AIDS, highlighting the consequences of idealizations of American childhood reveals both resistance and pain over the loss of children as well as a self-serving glorification of white childhood.

Race and class issues come into play in that poor children and children of color have not been historically associated with idealized images or fantasies of childhood innocence as have children who resemble Little Eva and Amanda Farrell. Those children who fall outside of the ideal are often ignored or their illnesses are used as evidence of the pathology of the mother and the group to which the child belongs. Kenneth Keniston addresses this double standard by posing a rhetorical question: If HIV infection had initially appeared in white middle-class girls "between the ages of two and fifteen . . . would the political response to AIDS have been the same as it has been in actuality?" (xxvii–xxviii). Clearly, as Keniston suggests, the response would have been very different if the first victim had been Little Eva instead of gay men and injection drug users, two groups whom many associate with perversion and debasement. American culture cherishes the idea of disease-free, innocent white female childhood and adolescence—even though it rarely addresses the actual complexities of girls and young women, whether they are outside the "privileged populations of industrialized states" or within it (Keniston, xxvii–xxviii).[3]

An outstanding theoretical exploration of AIDS, childhood innocence, and race comes not from a literary or cultural theorist but from a fiction writer and pediatrician named Perri Klass. Klass's novel, *Other Women's Children* (1990), focuses on the efficacy of sentimental literary and cultural forms when creating representations of childhood illness and death. As if conducting an inquiry into sentimental childhood, race, and AIDS and what happens when all three collide, Klass uses the novel format to intervene in the seemingly sympathetic culture of literary sentimentality. Her text considers the impact of idealized childhood on the bodies of the children and families who are not part of the normative ideal by focusing on children outside of what counts as innocent childhood. Klass contributes not only to an understanding of race and class in AIDS discourse on babies and children but to an understanding of literary sentimentality as a whole.

Other Women's Children is a stunning examination of the limits of the sentimental tradition as well as of its continuity. Similar to some feminist literary theory on the sentimental, such as the work of Laura Wexler and Lauren Berlant, Klass's novel interprets the sentimental paradigm as a form of unintentional cultural violence but also as inevitable. Throughout the text, Klass includes select passages from key canonical texts—*Little Women*, *The Old Curiosity Shop*, and, of course, *Uncle Tom's Cabin*—interpreted in terms of the AIDS epidemic, while also making clear that the sentimental cannot simply be discarded or denigrated. Using a pronounced postmodern sensibility, *Other Women's Children* questions the sentimental paradigm but also argues that to question it is not an escape from it, a theme that underscores the pervasiveness of the sentimental paradigm in representations of death, illness, and identity. The novel ends with idealized fantasies of domesticity, even though the chapters that precede it are full of angry critiques of sentimental novels. But the novel's most powerful contribution is its analysis of race and sentimentality.

Race, Sympathy, and the Child with AIDS

Using the subject of AIDS as a lens, *Other Women's Children* questions the entire project of sentimental literature of childhood death and illness. It is as if Klass's text were putting the sentimental literary tradition on trial.[4] Carefully organized around the life and thoughts of Amelia Stern, a devoted, overworked pediatrician, novelist, wife, and mother, the novel opens with Amelia's concern about one of her patients, Darren, a three-year-old African American boy with AIDS. Darren was orphaned by a mother who died of AIDS and has an absent father who is now exhibiting symptoms. He is cared for by his maternal grandmother, a worn-out retired schoolteacher named Roberta Wilson. Darren's days are filled with the stench of the hospital, terrifying medical procedures, and tantrums.

As a result of Amelia's contact with Darren, and her struggle to write a novel about the life of a writer-doctor-mother-wife, she begins a relentless analysis of some of her most cherished assumptions about childhood, justice, medicine, and sentimental literature. Klass skillfully balances a focus on the events in Amelia's life with Amelia's own investigation of literary children, for it is this interweaving of perspectives that leads to Amelia's insight: "Dying children are the sweet creamy centers of literature" (58).

Interspersed throughout the novel are Amelia's shrewd musings on the "uses" of children in nineteenth-century American and British literature. For instance, Amelia refers angrily to Beth March's famous deathbed scene in *Little Women*: "This chapter is pathos by the spoonful, this is the holy death of one too good to stay with us, whom the Almighty called to His bosom too soon. It is the whole damned nineteenth century, if you ask me" (63). Amelia feels frustrated by such literary models. As a doctor, she cannot save her young patients, in particular, young Darren; and as a writer, she cannot figure out how to tell the stories of her young patients without resorting to a recapitulation of the cherished sentimental texts of her childhood—texts she now finds problematic: "How can anyone write about children who get sick and die? What is most heart-piercing in life can turn into bathos, melodrama, sentimental nonsense in fiction" (8).

Klass's Amelia Stern is caught between her secure, happy childhood memories of reading *Uncle Tom's Cabin*, *Little Women*, and *The Old Curiosity Shop* and her observations that the ill children in her care are nothing like these literary "fictional angels" (203). For instance, when little Darren is placed in the intensive care unit, Amelia sarcastically reports to the reader: "He was very far from any gentle death scene I might have imagined for him, far from [Louisa May Alcott's] Beth [March] and far from [Harriet Beecher Stowe's] little Eva, far from every child who ever slipped quietly into the kind arms of death, its little arms too weak to hold the painful life any longer" (255).

Amelia continues to explore her feelings about the lives of her young patients, her love for her young, healthy son, and her thoughts about her husband in terms of her newfound skepticism and rage over nineteenth-century sentimental fiction. The more she analyzes these categories of her life, the more she begins to move beyond the typical complaint that sentimental discourses result in inferior literature and in obfuscation of the grim "realism" of death and dying. By the middle of the novel, Amelia adopts instead a cultural critique based not in theories of "realism" but in theories of race and class inequalities. That is, while Amelia continues to expose the gap between her actual experiences of childhood death and the representations of such deaths in literature, her most powerful insight concerns the race and class underpinnings of who gets to be the fictional angel in classic literature. Amelia rejects the view that sentimental discourses are simply unconvincing and instead adopts a critique of the material politics of Harriet Beecher Stowe's saintly Little Eva.

Klass argues that the reason Topsy does not die in *Uncle Tom's Cabin* is that she is "too bad to die"; she is not fit to teach moral lessons, to be an exemplar of womanhood, or to be a moral spokeswoman/mother of the nation. Topsy is a white-induced fantasy, and her body and history are irrelevant to the story. In comparing the life and dying of three-year-old Darren with that of Stowe's Little Eva, Amelia comes to the conclusion that fictional angels such as Little Eva rest upon the erasure of their racial and economic privilege. Amelia's analysis of *Uncle Tom's Cabin* uncovers the literary politics involved in decisions about whose emotionality gets represented and how, and whose emotionality is left out of representations and why. Klass's protagonist reveals racial and class superiority as the cornerstone, the central element, of the sentimental heroine.

For instance, in a key chapter titled "Has There Ever Been a Child like Eva," Amelia wonders why Little Eva, the well-cared-for child, dies, while the battered, malnourished servant/slave child, Topsy, escapes death. She concludes that the rhetorical excess and flourish of a sentimental death are the privilege of white Christian children:

> Topsy is surely statistically the child in that book who should not have lived to grow up, but then, can you imagine Topsy in that death scene? Topsy is too bad to die; she lies and steals and could not be presumed to be going straight to heaven. . . . One child will survive, but not the one who has every reason to—good food, medical attention, love and gentleness surrounding her. That one will die. (98)

Klass's text narrows in on "the battered, beaten, overworked and undernourished" Topsy in contrast to the refined, saintly Little Eva in an effort to lay open the racial superiority that bolsters the sentimental child (98). Such a juxtaposition makes clear how Little Eva's spectacular death is constructed against the denial of Topsy's abused nine-year-old body.

In explaining to his cousin, Miss Ophelia, how he came to purchase Topsy, Mr. St. Clare (Eva's father) says that Topsy "belonged to a couple of drunken creatures that keep a low restaurant that I have to pass every day, and I was tired of hearing her screaming, and them beating and screaming at her" (Stowe, 354). According to Patricia A. Turner, Stowe's allusion here to severe physical and emotional abuse is rooted in historical accuracy. Turner writes, "Historical documents offer ample evidence that from the era of slavery to the present, many black children have been underclothed, overworked, underfed, and safer in the company of animals than with some human beings" (16). Although Stowe knew the "particulars of . . . a neglected, abused child" such as Topsy, her text rationalizes why it must be silent on these "particulars": "[I]n this world, multitudes must live and die in a state that it would be too great a shock to the nerves of their fellow-mortals even to hear described" (355). In other words, Topsy's experiences are unspeakable.

Such a response regarding the "particulars" of Topsy's life is intriguing. Topsy is but eight years old. She has been surrounded by sadistic racists and possibly psychotics; she has never been educated or allowed to grow and develop. Her former living conditions were most likely unsanitary; she wore dirty clothes, was malnourished, and was subjected to repeated physical beatings and mental abuse. And yet Stowe repeatedly alludes to

Topsy's abuse only to wipe it out. Instead, Stowe depicts Topsy as a physically energetic trickster who breaks into dance at the drop of a hat and performs one mischievous trick after another. Eva's father summons Topsy by "giving a whistle, as a man would to call the attention of a dog" and makes his request: "Give us a song, now, and show us some of your dancing" (352).

In other words, Stowe evokes the physical and emotional details of abuse of children under slavery in order to bolster her overall argument that slavery is anti-Christian and antifamily; but then she trivializes Topsy's brutal experiences by constructing her as an empty-headed entertainer. Stowe also belittles Topsy's experiences by glorifying the character of Little Eva. The denial of Topsy's body is the flip side of the etherealization and spiritualization of Little Eva's.

While Eva is described as graceful, fragile, and relentlessly "otherworldly," Topsy is described as a "glittering serpent" (364). Topsy's animalistic physicality is further developed when Stowe refers to her as "goblin-like," "heathenish," "a monkey," a cat, and a bat (351, 352, 365). Yet for all Topsy's gross physicality, for all of her animalistic embodiment and "carnival of confusion," the actual physical realities of her life are ignored (366). Topsy escapes the death reserved for privileged girls like Eva because Topsy is just not good enough for sentimental transcendence. Her lying and stealing, behaviors St. Clare assumes she picked up in her deplorable life with the speculators, offend everyone, except, of course, Little Eva. Under Eva's tutorship, the "heathenish" goblin Topsy converts to white Christianity, making clear that the only childhood worth emulating and grieving over is Eva's.[5]

Klass's Amelia Stern, however, wants to know what actually exists behind the stereotyped Topsy. As a doctor and writer, Amelia wants to know more about Topsy's bodily health and life circumstances, and by wanting to know the material details, Amelia is once again suggesting the underlying ideology of white superiority in *Uncle Tom's Cabin* as well as in updated versions of the famous novel. Klass makes clear that producing tears and sympathy in readers through the figure of the idealized white child is not the same as producing critical reflection. In fact, Klass's novel actively resists what Lauren Berlant calls "citation of the *Uncle Tom* form" (639). Berlant argues, similar to Klass, that "the forces of distortion in the world of feeling politics put into play by the citation of *Uncle Tom* are as likely to justify ongoing forms of domination as to give form and language to impulses toward resistance" (640).

Klass's text boldly uses the novel form to promote a critical view that can be applied to any interpretation of children and AIDS. From Amelia Stern's skeptical standpoint, Hoffman's Amanda Farrell is an updated Little Eva, a child who, statistically speaking, is the least likely to die of AIDS. This skepticism allows the reader to wonder how many lives and deaths are hidden behind the spectacle of Amanda Farrell's death, just as Topsy's body is hidden behind the white spectacle of Little Eva. While Stowe, Hoffman, and Klass all focus on illness in children, they do so with very different goals in mind.

Other Women's Children participates in an established, ongoing critical dialogue on the sentimental paradigm by challenging, resisting, and questioning what it means to construct sentimental AIDS. But Klass's novel also reveals the impossibility of ever moving beyond a "postsentimental" paradigm.[6] Although her text resists an uncritical "*Uncle Tom* form," her character's struggle reminds us of the power of the form itself as well as its enmeshment in national rhetoric. The fictionalized argument that the privileging of Eva's death is an erasure of the lived complexities of Topsy's history and body is expressed in a self-reflexive, postmodern style, one that expresses desire for the very paradigm the novel sets out to critique. In this way, *Other Women's Children* moves beyond denigration on the one hand or uncritical sanctification on the other by showing the protagonist's attraction to and embeddedness in the form as well as her repulsion and resistance.[7] *Other Women's Children* not only raises questions about whose tears and whose emotionality organize the sentimental paradigm but suggests the centrality of the sentimental paradigm into the late twentieth century and beyond.

However, like many narratives on HIV, Klass's ignores the implications of how the dying child in AIDS discourse interacts with representations and material realities of women. In *Other Women's Children*, the needs of the ill child consistently overshadow the needs of adult women. I find this a powerful contradiction, not an aesthetic or political flaw. Klass's contradictory stance on women in relation to the sentimental child unwittingly makes intelligible the degree to which even progressive, critical conversations about sentimental AIDS depend upon traditional paradigms of gender.

Babies, HIV, and Motherhood

When traditional sacrificial motherhood—as opposed to feminist mothering or other oppositional models of motherhood—intersects with the discourse of baby HIV, the resulting language and imagery of women are very disturbing. The subsumption of the mother by the child is part of the motif of the good woman as romanticized, passive, selfless mother, a cultural belief that is firmly implanted in medical research, practice, and literary responses to AIDS. This entrenched idea of woman/mother influences all aspects of women's health, from prevention to treatment to research. For example, it is still common for federally funded researchers, medical practitioners, and the media to speak about women's health in terms of how it affects other people—namely, fetuses, babies, children, and men (Corea, 40–51). The few research studies designed for women and AIDS in the 1980s were designated as "Pediatric AIDS" and "The Prostitute Study"—hence, the bad mother and the whore (Corea, 44, 49). Unfortunately, not much has changed since then.

Mainstream news, medical research, fiction, film, and television continue to reinforce the idea that pediatric AIDS is synonymous with women's health, and that the mother's health is simply an aspect of the health of children. At the 1998 International AIDS Conference in Geneva "most of the presentations addressed perinatal transmission only, with little attention to the health needs of the mother" (Denison, "Pregnancy and Perinatal Transmission," 6). Mother-to-child transmission, or perinatal HIV transmission, is a vital area of AIDS research with benefits for women, their babies, and their families and communities. But researchers and writers need to look beyond perinatal transmission and gynecological concerns. Both of these areas of women's health are important in treating HIV disease, but they are not the only areas in which HIV disease manifests in women (Averit, "New Studies Show Why," 4).

For example, for all its rebelliousness and insights on race, Klass's novel reproduces the idea that women's health is synonymous with children's by ignoring the effects of idealized dying children and AIDS discourses on representations of women's experiences and health. *Other Women's Children* examines the racism of sentimental AIDS in terms of children, but Klass's text, ironically, privileges the narrative of the child over the rights, needs, and health of women. In her memoir, *Baby Doctor: A Pediatrician's*

Training, Klass continues to express her skepticism about sentimentality through a series of nonfiction vignettes on HIV-infected children who range in age from one to eight and a half years old. Shadowy references to infected family members and caretakers appear, too, but as in her novel, sick children and how to represent them are Klass's focus.[8]

As in her novel, Klass questions whether sentimental representations of children and AIDS are "useful": "These children, and their families, represent an enormous need. To take care of them properly requires not just sympathy, hugs, and tears, but money and extensive medical and social services" (*Baby Doctor,* 196–97). But in both Klass's memoir and her novel, the perspectives and experiences of adult women are incidental. It is natural that Klass as a pediatrician would focus on children and that she would write a novel and a nonfiction book that privilege the child. Even physicians who are not pediatricians find the death of a child harder to take than the death of an adult.

In her review of *Other Women's Children,* Vanessa Northington Gamble recounts her first autopsy of a child: "I remember thinking that the child was out of place. He did not belong in this cold, sterile room. He should have been outside playing" (11). Gamble became so upset "seeing the blond boy lying on the table" that she had to leave the morgue (11). But feelings of immense sorrow do not cancel out the need to reflect on a cultural pattern that places children's health and deaths against women's. *Other Women's Children* nourishes this paradigm by constructing Amelia Stern as a selfless martyr, which draws comment from Gamble: Klass's Amelia "reminds me how often women ignore their own needs and how often medical professionals are reluctant to seek help" (11). The practice of putting the child before the mother/woman is not beneficial to mother or child. Rebecca Denison, an HIV-positive mother, activist, and writer, argues that a mother whose health is treated as a priority is better able to care for a child; in addition, her health is often better if she is not caring for a sick child. In ignoring adult women and AIDS and in presenting Amelia Stern as an isolated martyr, Klass reproduces one of the major barriers to women's access to health care.[9] Women's infection, if it is mentioned at all, counts only in terms of its effects on others—namely, children.

For instance, Klass writes in *Baby Doctor:* "As more women are infected with the virus, pediatric cases of AIDS are becoming increasingly common" (189). Again, while I do not want to downplay the suffering of children and their parents, my point is that Klass's focus on children at the expense of women contributes to the conceptualization of women as mere conduits of either infection or selfless care to infants and men.

Other Women's Children does explore women's conflicts between paid work and unpaid work in the home; in her focus on Amelia Stern's competing roles as a pediatrician and as a mother and wife, this theme is dramatized. However, she does not allow her character to explore women's conflicting roles with the same level of critical acumen that Amelia displays in her race and class analysis of innocent childhood. The same depth and intensity with which Amelia launches her critique of the sentimental deaths of literary children are not applied to the conflicts in Amelia's own life. For instance, by the end of the novel, Amelia's husband, Matt, leaves her (he takes their son with him but eventually the family is reunited) because he feels she put the needs of "other women's children" before the less dramatic—but still most important—needs of their son. Amazingly, Klass then has Amelia "repent" for her supposed motherly negligence of her son rather than explain to her husband that he too needs to learn how to parent. An unexplored tension in this novel is that even a female character as "exceptional" as Klass's Amelia Stern cannot escape the expectations of sacrificial woman.

Akin to the traditional sentimental heroine, Amelia Stern must work alone, "as a one-woman unit" (A. Douglas, *Feminization*, 157). Amelia has no community of doctors, activists, and feminists, who might study the issues of gender and the medical profession, as well as the connections among race, class, AIDS, medical ethics, and health care. In fact, collective action is ridiculed in Amelia's satirical characterization of political activists, especially her mother. Amelia sees her mother as a naive "do-gooder" who never finished her academic degree in social work and who has spent much of her adult life surrounding herself with "fringe" people. Ambivalent and contemptuous toward her mother's low-status work in a soup kitchen, Amelia fails to see her own self-sacrificing, do-gooder practices.

Klass's apparent inability to free her protagonist from the gendered mandate of solitary, self-sacrificing caretaking is a powerful and compelling contradiction paralleling Amelia's unacknowledged ambivalence about abolishing a sentimental view of women as self-sacrificing, domestic angels. In this way, Klass's text retreats from the very analysis she initiates, providing the reader with a contradictory text that is both postsentimental and sentimental at the same time. As the good woman, Amelia is able to critique the sentimental discourses that she has found emotionally nourishing throughout her life only if to do so will somehow help sick children. On behalf of disadvantaged children, she will face and perhaps relinquish her need for and dependency on literary spiritualized death. On behalf of adult women, however, Klass's text has little to say.

Tellingly, in *Baby Doctor* Klass states that when attending a birth she is always more interested in the child's health than in the mother's: "Though I have myself been in the position of the mother, though I identify with women in labor and now often do find myself pushing along with them till my muscles ache, as soon as there is a baby in the room, I lose any medical interest in the mother. Given a choice between an adult and a child, I prefer to take care of the child" (240). Unfortunately, her preference for infants and children seems to be the choice American medicine has made as well, as many documents and studies indicate.

Klass's text exposes the effects of sentimental discourses on representations of HIV-infected poor children and poor children of color, but pulls back from doing this same sort of work on the representations of adult women with HIV/AIDS. Yet the connection among women's subordination, gendered status, and the racialized sentimental paradigm is also part of what is oppressive about sentimental discourses.

TV Mothers and AIDS

> Television is, quite simply, the most powerful cultural
> form in history. What it tells us about the world is, for
> most people, what is taken for reality.
> Elayne Rapping, "You've Come Which Way, Baby?"

Women's health is also undermined by the figure of woman as the dangerous, irresponsible baby killer who infects her child. In direct contrast to woman as conduit of sacrifice, redemption, and moral instruction, this conception of the bad mother as the conduit of selfishness and death circulates in various venues, including media reports, medical research, and network television. Two 1999 CNN reports on AIDS exemplify the transformation of women's lived complexities into moral statements about HIV-positive women's supposed irresponsibility. One report, "Women and AIDS: The Forgotten Epidemic," presents itself as a challenge to women's invisibility, but the portrait of women and AIDS that emerges is all too familiar:

> [T]hese drug-abusing women are often having unprotected sex with men who share needles with others. And even if the women are not themselves having sex with multiple partners, the men in their lives may well be— leading to an elaborate, increasingly risky chain reaction through which HIV and other sexually transmitted diseases are transmitted in all directions.

The women (and men) are described as a collective "chain" of infection spreading disease "in all directions," and their exposure is based on reckless behavior. What medical research knows about HIV in women's bodies, what information it has on how women can protect themselves, and what theories it has about why some men refuse to use condoms (this last topic is rarely addressed by medical authorities at national and international conferences) are never mentioned.[10] Instead, the report constructs women as chaotic channels of infection involved with wild, destructive men.

Another CNN report, published a few weeks later, announces a major breakthrough in baby HIV and includes statements by Dr. Anthony Fauci of the National Institutes of Health. The good news—and it is good news—is that a drug called nevirapine dramatically reduces perinatal transmission and costs only $4 a dose. However, the only mention of adult women is, again, as mediums of transmission. In addition, although the nevirapine study was conducted in Uganda, Fauci invokes American women, whom he describes as "frustrating":

> [Nevirapine] might come in handy . . . when people come into a clinic or emergency room not having any prenatal care whatsoever, and they come in just about to go into labor. . . .
>
> You won't be in a frustrating situation of saying, "My goodness, you should have come in 25 weeks ago or 30 weeks ago when you first knew you were pregnant."

Since there is no discussion of or investigation into why HIV-positive women do not receive prenatal care, Fauci creates the impression that HIV-positive American women simply do not have the human decency to take care of their unborn children. While women who use illegal drugs are least likely to have prenatal care, many of these women either do not know that they are HIV-positive or are afraid to disclose for fear of losing their children (Denison, "Pregnancy and Perinatal Transmission," 7).

HIV-positive women's motherhood as toxic to the nation and family is embedded in the made-for-television film *A Place for Annie* (1994), a striking example of a "bad woman/mother" in a fictionalized AIDS narrative. Mary-Louise Parker assumes the role of Linda Marsten, a white, unemployed injection drug user and mother who gives birth to an HIV-positive baby. In this drama, the HIV-positive woman is the epitome of selfish, pathological American motherhood.

The film opens in the pediatric intensive care unit of a hospital where Susan Lansing, a pediatric intensive care nurse played by Sissy Spacek, scolds a colleague for not taking proper care of nine-week-old Annie Marsten, the HIV-positive baby Linda abandoned. It is clear that the employee is uncomfortable with the infected baby and that this scene is meant to emphasize the theme of stigma. Alice, the hospital's African American social worker, is trying to place Annie in an adopted family, but "nobody wants her." Susan learns that Annie is going to be transferred to Tremont State Hospital, a grim, decrepit place full of doomed children waiting to die. Divorced with a teenage son, Susan decides she is going to adopt Annie, even though the social worker tries to dissuade her. David, Susan's son, is also against the idea. Nevertheless, Susan paints and wallpapers the baby's room and hires a nanny.

The climax of the first act occurs when Linda Marsten tries to regain custody of Annie, who is now living a comfortable life in Susan's suburban home. Linda is in recovery and she wants her daughter back. In Linda's first appearance on the television screen, she's angry, agitated, and she parades through the social worker's office wearing a miniskirt, a low-cut, tight-fitting blouse, and high heels. A chain smoker, she constantly holds a lit cigarette and chews gum. From the start, the viewer is encouraged to see that this female character is bad, and her inevitable death from AIDS will not be presented, step-by-step, with visitations from angels, but instead as the punishment she deserves. At one point in the film, Linda emphasizes this point when she tells her baby daughter, "I deserve what's gonna happen to me. You don't."

Susan responds to Linda's custody suit with anger: "I'm going to fight you on this." The judge grants Linda visitation rights, and Susan explodes in the social worker's office: "She's a drug addict. She's got AIDS." Keeping true to character, irresponsible Linda brings Annie home late and Susan hurls one insult after another, calling Linda an "airhead junkie" who is "so brain dead from drugs you can't even tell time." Furious that Annie will be taken away from her, Susan comes up with a better plan: she asks Linda to move into her home, so that they can all be a family. "You'll have a home," Susan tells Linda. She entices Linda with the promise of free medical care and drugs, although we never know how Susan can accomplish this. Linda, presumably because she has no integrity left and no practical options, moves into Susan's teenage son's room, and proceeds to anger and annoy every member of the family, including the nanny and baby Annie, who often cries in her biological mother's presence. Linda flicks her cigarette ash into David's aquarium, falls asleep with a lit cigarette and sets the mattress on fire, ignores her daughter, and fails to notice when the child is playing with matches. After each unmotherly and careless act, Susan screams: "What is wrong with you?"

What is wrong with Linda is that she is the victim of bad mothering as well as the practitioner of bad mothering. When Linda calls her mother to tell her about her health, the mother hangs up. Only at the end of the second act, when Linda is clearly dying, do she and Susan begin to create a friendship and alternative family. Slowly, the household begins to open up to Linda. The nanny, who once made it clear that she was working for Susan and Annie's sake, "not for *her*," begins to soften toward Linda and encourages the dying mother to feed Annie. Susan's entire household has been determined to keep the pathological Linda away from Annie, but now that Linda is approaching death, they embrace her and teach her the beauty of the mother-child bond.

In act 3, Linda leaves Susan's house to die in an AIDS hospice—a taxi picks her up so Susan's family won't be inconvenienced. Before going to the hospice, Linda gives Susan some good news: she has legally given her custody of Annie. "You're such a good person. You're such a good mother," says Linda. Later, Susan learns that Annie has shed her mother's immune system and is no longer testing positive for HIV, and she rushes to Linda's deathbed to tell her before she dies: "You didn't give her death. You gave her life."

The theme of female unity and maternal sacrifice as a universal force gradually replaces the mistrust and judgmental attitudes that have kept Susan and Linda in bitter conflict. Good and bad mother unite over what is best for Annie, and because they have both been abandoned by their own parents—Susan because she got divorced, and Linda because she comes from the classic, low-class, "bad" family—they forge an unlikely yet intense friendship. Despite their reconciliation, *A Place for Annie* ends with the message that getting a baby away from a bad mother and into the hands of a good mother is the moral response to perinatal transmission and infected mothers. Linda's character reinforces the myth of the poorly educated, out-of-control, unemployed woman; Linda's health is incidental to the health and well-being of the baby, and her death is her redemption for the sin of being a bad mother/woman. The myth of the poor woman as reckless, infectious womb is left intact, and the myth of white, innocent childhood is preserved.

The Good White Mother, Welfare Queens, and AIDS

Linda Marsten's mothering in *A Place for Annie* is portrayed as the inevitable result of her being a poor, unemployed welfare mother who fails to rise above her unfortunate circumstances. In fact, her characterization crystallizes a connection between the creation and dismantling of the welfare state and the discourse of women and AIDS. Such a comparison rests on the figure of the idealized mother. This figure rationalizes (and demands) women's unpaid caregiving as it uses the good woman as a benchmark for what counts as the ideal American citizen—white, heterosexual, a mother, and married. Lesser citizens, or those perceived to be of low moral character (such as Linda Marsten), can be rehabilitated through the educational mission of the good mother; if not, they do not deserve to be seen as mothers and they do not deserve state provision, as the recent welfare reform policies imply. Just as "lesser" women are being created and then denigrated in the restructuring of welfare, women with HIV/AIDS who cannot emulate an updated version of the good mother/suffering woman are similarly chastised.

The attack on poor women's "bad" mothering in debates on welfare reform speaks to the fact that no other figure is more central to American politics than the maternal woman. A seemingly apolitical figure, the good mother operates as an allegorical female who preserves the national character and epitomizes compassionate democracy. Held up as both a bulwark against moral decay and a guide for the wayward and the outcast, this figure is central in American myths, histories, and political struggles. She serves a pivotal role in the creation of the American welfare state and, as I have been arguing, in promoting a "compassionate" (although problematic) discourse on AIDS.

According to Gwendolyn Mink, the contemporary American welfare state is rooted in the nineteenth- and early-twentieth-century concept of white, middle-class motherhood as the salvation of the nation.[11] Since early democracy equated male citizenship with a public, political project, female citizenship had to be figured as an educational, moral mission, as an application of mothering on a national scale. In this way, Anglo-Saxon middle-class women, while lacking full political, economic, and civil rights, became an expression of what Mink calls "white men's democracy" and the white man's ideal American character (372).

The Anglo-Saxon citizen-mother was the ideal against which all other citizens could be judged: lesser men and women, new immigrants, blacks, the poor. White motherhood was responsible not only for the nation's moral future through the reproduction of the good heterosexual family / citizen, but also for the resolution of elite white male anxieties over racial and ethnic diversity brought about by immigration, urbanization, and industrialization. Elite men's typical response to people or events they perceived as threats was to exclude and/or place restrictions on cultural practices not associated with the founding fathers. Reform-minded women typically responded to perceived threats with assimilation, compassionate democracy, and educational reform.

Thus the good mother uplifted suspect Americans, making them fit for citizenship and soothing elite men's fears over introducing racially and ethnically diverse people into the political community. Similarly, public discourse on AIDS also evokes the concept of threat to the nation and denounces people with AIDS as questionable citizens. At the same time, a parallel public discourse has denounced this view and has served to instruct Americans on how to incorporate the person with AIDS into the national imagination. The figure of the caring white mother is essential to this project.

The moral role of the mother gave acceptable women access to the state and to political change in women's terms. As Mink argues, it was in this historical and political context that women argued that the husbandless citizen-mother deserved state money in order to fulfill her duty to the nation. In order for promising mothers to rise above low morals and emulate the ideal mother, they had to be kept out of waged work and receive state aid for their children.

Thus, dependency in "salvageable" women was acceptable since these same women could be taught to reproduce citizens worthy of America. On the other hand, dependency in men was seen as slavish and feminine; dependency in "unsalvageable women," that is, in women who could never be rehabilitated, was interpreted as further evidence of the women's unworthiness. "Unsalvageable" women either were denied assistance or had their assistance taken away.

The idea then as now is that some women are fit for motherhood and some are not; some women's mothering counts and deserves financial support and some women's mothering does not. It is this underlying belief that fueled the dismantling of Aid to Families with Dependent Children (AFDC), a campaign that began in the 1980s under the Reagan Administration and was completed by Bill Clinton in 1996 with the passage of the Personal Responsibility and Work Opportunity Reconciliation Act (PRWORA). At the same time that single mothers on welfare were being stereotyped as lazy, incompetent, bad mothers who bred children in order to get more money, heterosexual, married, middle-class women were being urged to leave the paid labor market and nurture their husbands and children instead. Critics asserted that the breakdown of the two-parent family was the cause of welfare, and that by ending welfare the state would actually be saving the family by encouraging women to marry men. Charles S. Murray, the controversial co-author of *The Bell Curve*, argued for the complete dismantling of welfare rather than its proposed transformation from AFDC to TANF, Temporary Assistance to Needy Families. Murray's solution to the problem of poverty was plain and simple: heterosexual marriage. So while heterosexual marriage was being promoted as the answer to the crisis of poverty in families, poor mothers with children were cast as breeders of damaged children.

The state essentially told poor women that they should return to the paid labor market because their claim to motherhood was not authentic. Transformed from bad welfare mothers into "providers," most able-bodied poor women are now being funneled into low-paying service jobs. As Heather McCallum explains, "Women are expected to act as fathers, providing economically for their families" (57). Thus, the so-called welfare queen evoked by President Reagan in the 1980s is beyond redemption and assimilation into the good mother-citizen role. The welfare mother, as constructed by patriarchy and white supremacy, has absolutely nothing to offer America, and her mothering and caretaking are a joke; as an unfit mother, her caregiving work is invisible, and she is used instead to provide cheap labor for an expanding service economy. In the discourse of welfare and welfare reform, all poor women, especially poor black women and women of color, are suspect; in the discourse of AIDS, these same women, along with infected queers and drug users, fall outside the national family.

Real Mothers with HIV and AIDS

A solid example of work on mothering and morality that is "strategically negotiating between engrained codes of maternity and embracing the lived complexities of chosen motherhood" is W.O.R.L.D. (Liss, 82). W.O.R.L.D., an organization of and for women with HIV infection, generates an ongoing, evolving, dynamic discourse on women and AIDS, including a complex view of mothering, perinatal transmission, and mother/child treatment. This latter focus, however, has stirred some controversy among readers.

In 1997, readers wrote to Rebecca Denison, the editor of the organization's newsletter, and complained about the increased focus on mother-to-child transmission. Many HIV-infected women and women with AIDS do not have children and are not planning to get pregnant, and these readers resented the linkage of women's health with children's health. Dension, an HIV-positive mother of twins, responded to the complaints by pointing out that "HIV+ moms and children are part of our community. So we suggest to those who are put off, don't read it" ("Pediatric AIDS," 5).

What is very impressive about W.O.R.L.D.'s newsletter, including the articles on pediatric AIDS and perinatal transmission, is that it always includes a pronounced awareness of how women are socialized to put the needs of the baby before their own as well as an awareness of how dominant institutions validate this behavior. There are repeated assertions that empower HIV-positive women to claim their right to health care: "Many women have difficulty making their own health a priority when they have a baby and/or others to care for" (Denison, "New Guidelines," 4); "Those women who want to limit the baby's exposure to HIV drugs could choose to take AZT alone, but should know that this is not the best choice for their own health" (Denison, "New Guidelines," 5). And my favorite: "Pregnancy should not be used as an excuse to deny or delay offering [a woman] the same treatments as would be offered to a person who is not pregnant" (Denison, "New Guidelines," 4). There is nothing troubling about a focus on perinatal transmission in a women's newsletter, as long as the focus on pregnancy and transmission does not encourage the medical establishment to use women's pregnancy against them.

W.O.R.L.D. consistently addresses the social constructions of gender in the medical community—and society at large—that make HIV-positive women feel they are not "mommy material."[12] This view of HIV-positive women is what makes the issue of AIDS and pregnancy of concern to all feminists, whether they have children or not: the devaluation of mother is the devaluation of women. A positive woman's decision to have a child, despite the disapproval of authorities and community, is daring because the woman is expressing the right to her own body as well as to a chosen motherhood. Terry McGovern argues that debates surrounding HIV-positive women and reproduction "are squarely within *Roe v. Wade* territory" (quoted in Farber, 58).

Women who are HIV-positive and pregnant are subject to a multitude of coercive behaviors. In the eighties, they were both coerced into having abortions and sometimes denied access to abortions (Corea, 47). Today, they are expected to take AZT to prevent perinatal transmission even though some women cannot tolerate AZT and even though there is still not enough research on the long-term effects of AZT on the child, especially as the child reaches adolescence and adulthood (Farber, 53–65).[13] Women are also encouraged to discontinue combination drug therapy— which is the standard of care for adults—because no one knows the effects of protease inhibitors on the fetus; if they choose to remain on pro-

tease inhibitors for their own health, they are seen as endangering the fetus. In other words, discontinuing drug therapy may prove beneficial to
the fetus—although there is little research to support this claim one way
or the other—and yet discontinuing combination therapy puts the
woman's health at risk. Rebecca Denison's view on these difficult decisions is that all women should have the right to choose and that more
complex research on pregnant women and AIDS is needed. A woman
should be allowed to choose whether to discontinue combination therapy—a danger to her because she may develop resistance to the antiviral
drugs—or to continue using protease inhibitors. Whether one is a mother
or not, the right of women to make decisions about their bodies, health,
and treatment is of concern to all citizens. State control of women's bodies, as evidenced by calls for mandatory testing of all pregnant women, is
a danger for all.[14]

Rhetoric calling for mandatory testing of pregnant women and mandatory AZT to prevent perinatal transmission is ironic since the actual treatment of some babies born to infected mothers suggests widespread indifference. Klass's *Other Women's Children* proposes that while the dominant
culture clings to the notion of innocent white childhood, it does little to en-
sure that each child, whether HIV-infected or not, has access to health
care.[15] For instance, Amelia Stern's anguish stems in part from understanding the stark differences of care given to her son and the poor "clinic
children" she treats. However Rebecca Denison, white, middle-class, and
married, reports that she and her child were (mis)treated by health care
workers because of her "history":

> I took Sophia to the emergency room of a children's hospital on a Friday
> night with a high fever. From 10:30 PM to 4:30 AM, she was stuck with nee-
> dles over a dozen times, with little regard for her pain. During the lumbar
> puncture, the woman who held her down directed the guy doing the pro-
> cedure, which failed after three sticks. When I told the physician in charge
> that I didn't want any more students practicing on my child, she ignored
> me and instead said she was diagnosing my child with pneumonia, "based
> on your history." (She thought she had AIDS). . . . Later I was told, "Sophia
> doesn't have pneumonia after all." (Diaz and Denison, "What We Learned
> the Hard Way," 6)

Denison's story, and many others published by W.O.R.L.D., show that the denigration of HIV-positive women, even ones with "acceptable" race and class credentials, is prevalent and interferes with the actual care of babies. Maintaining the myth of innocent childhood is more important to the public than the actual lives of infected babies and the women who are their mothers. Concepts of sanctified motherhood and innocent childhood undermine actual mothering.

CHAPTER 4

THE LESBIAN MAMMY

> Blanche was unimpressed by the tears, and Grace's
> Mammy-save-me eyes. Mammy-savers regularly
> peeped out at her from the faces of some white women
> for whom she worked. . . . She never ceased to be
> amazed at how many white people longed for Aunt
> Jemima. They'd ease into the kitchen and hem and haw
> their way through some sordid personal tale. She'd lis-
> ten and make sympathetic noises.
>
> Barbara Neely, *Blanche on the Lam*

> The black female's body needs less to be rescued from
> the masculine "gaze" than to be sprung from a historic
> script surrounding her with signification while at the
> same time, and not paradoxically, it erases her com-
> pletely.
>
> Lorraine O'Grady, "Olympia's Maid:
> Reclaiming Black Female Subjectivity"

Blanche White, the protagonist of Barbara Neely's award-winning mystery novel *Blanche on the Lam*, is a middle-aged, black domestic worker whose opinions of her employer, Grace, are expressed throughout the book. Well aware of the construction of the black woman as "mammy" and "Aunt Jemima," Blanche humorously exposes what film historian Donald Bogle calls the enduring fantasy of "black women as nurturing, caretaking marvels . . . helping poor white women untangle the knots in their lives" (358–59).[1] Blanche pretends to "listen and make sympathetic noises," but readers know her true feelings of contempt and dislike, feelings that only increase as the story progresses, revealing that Grace is a psychotic killer (Neely, 39).

Neely's Blanche "performs" the role of mammy out of economic necessity, but this never stops her from having her own mind and life.[2] In fact, Blanche's insightful critical commentary on "mammy-save-me eyes" suggests how the production of tears functions as a smokescreen behind which lie the complex struggles and rage of African American women. Blanche's standpoint serves as a powerful angle of vision through which to examine representations of and silences on African American women and HIV in terms of white women's tears.[3] It makes visible the emergence of the newly created role of the "lesbian mammy" as a device for addressing the still stigmatized topic of AIDS.

Self-abnegation and selflessness—trademarks of the mammy as well as the "good white woman"—have unique implications in terms of women and AIDS. They are gender and race formulations that exacerbate women's risk of infection since they wipe out a sense of "self" whose health needs protection and attention. Unfortunately, AIDS and "the mammy" collide in one of the first Hollywood films to address women and AIDS, Herbert Ross's *Boys on the Side.* In this film, a nonthreatening, desexualized African American lesbian character serves as a white heterosexual fantasy that eases the dominant culture's fear of black female sexuality, lesbian sexuality, and AIDS. In an effort to temper this potent web of stigma, *Boys* focuses on a black woman who cares for a white, heterosexual, middle-class, HIV-positive woman. One crucial result of such a framework is that the impact of AIDS on the material lives of women of color is strategically erased and displaced onto white women.

In order to fully understand the construction of the lesbian mammy I want to explore the politics of sexuality and race in commercial films on AIDS.[4] My goal in analyzing Hollywood's response to AIDS is not to dismiss commercial films as trivial or lacking in artistic skill, or to denigrate the importance of the emotional outlet and visual pleasure film provides the spectator. *Boys* is a cultural narrative of competing political and aesthetic strands; it both resists and conforms to traditional racial and gender roles for women.

The social and economic meanings of the film may be teased out of its sentimentalized racial, gender, and sexual ideas of feminism, black lesbians, and AIDS. It is a cruel irony that although "[t]hree-fourths of women with AIDS are women of color," the one (and to my knowledge, only) commercial film on women and AIDS organizes the story around the classic figure of the suffering white woman (Denison, "Understanding,"

4). This interpretation of the film is not meant as moral chastisement of white women or feminism; rather it illustrates how the white female body is symbolically used to mediate destabilizing social stigmas such as AIDS. Such a practice transforms HIV-positive white women's experiences and bodies into a useful symbolism that erases, not only the realities and contradictions of HIV-positive white women's lives, but the very fact of HIV and AIDS in African American women.[5]

Yet the film is a potential source of pleasure for an audience/spectator. Although the racial and gender traditions coded in the narrative's sentimentality inevitably overwhelm the film, few people with personal experience of AIDS would easily reject discourses that allow people with AIDS and those who love them some narrative release and identification. A different text, *The Whispers of Angels,* includes many of the same conventions as *Boys* but incorporates into its aesthetic practice an analysis of the problematic use of sentimentality in representations of AIDS.

AIDS and Hollywood

The American studio system is unabashedly committed to high profit above all else, and any theme or social issue that frustrates this goal is often dismissed.[6] Yet, throughout its history, Hollywood has consistently (and problematically) addressed social, historical, and political themes in commercial films. Slavery, interracial relationships, economic depressions, human addictions, incest, and the Holocaust, to name some of the more obvious topics, have all been transformed into products of mass culture. In addition, the studio system itself has been the subject of books, articles, documentaries, and feature films as writers, film historians, scholars, and filmmakers plumb the significance of the products and practices of one of the most influential industries of the twentieth century.

Cultural critics and film historians look to commercial films for clues to how the dominant culture responds to and makes sense of social and historical controversies. As one might suspect, the story of AIDS and Hollywood is replete with silences, indifference, discrimination, and great reluctance. But pressure from the lesbian and gay community and from within the industry forced executives—both gay and straight—to finally make a film on AIDS. Although the epidemic officially began in 1981 and became, by the late 1980s, a global crisis, it was only in 1993 that Tristar Pictures released *Philadelphia,* the first Hollywood film to address the epidemic in America. In 1995 Warner Brothers released the first film to address AIDS in women, *Boys on the Side.*

I watched both of these films with a mixture of emotional neediness and intellectual skepticism. As someone craving public images of the devastating impact of AIDS on diverse Americans, I went with a need to be comforted, but I also understood that any film created to generate money and pity would undoubtedly disappoint. The convergence of AIDS and the commercial film industry's ethos of celebrity and profit resulted in film narratives that were safe, condescending, and burdened by unexamined assumptions about gay personhood and race. Nevertheless, *Philadelphia* and *Boys on the Side* are keenly significant to film criticism and history for the cultural frameworks they provide on AIDS and the taboo topics associated with it. In *Reel to Real: Race, Sex, and Class at the Movies,* bell hooks writes that "[m]ovies do not merely offer us the opportunity to reimagine the culture we most intimately know on the screen, they make culture" (9).

What the politics and aesthetics of these two films suggest is that narratives on AIDS are not "lies" so much as alterations of experiences that are too complex and dark for the conventions of most commercial films. The crucial question is not "What is an 'accurate' representation of AIDS?" but rather "What can we learn about culture when the complex viewpoints, feelings, and experiences engendered by AIDS are excised, altered, converted, and transformed into narratives that are rife with vague generalities and empty universalisms?

In many ways *Philadelphia* is one more example of a self-serving story created by the dominant, white heterosexual culture, this time by portraying a gay man who is saved by a reformed homophobic lawyer. Andrew Beckett (played by Tom Hanks) is a paradox, a white gay man both without a gay community and with one. In a large city with a viable gay community, he ostensibly cannot find a gay lawyer willing to buck the system. So he turns to a straight lawyer, Joe Miller (played by Denzel Washington), who heroically rids himself of homophobia and wins Beckett his civil rights. Throughout, Beckett insists he is "not political." But meanwhile, members of Philadelphia's gay community, including ACT-UP, come to his defense by protesting outside the courthouse.

Andrew Beckett is a highly paid corporate lawyer in a powerful, old-money law firm. He exists in a largely white, upper-middle-class, professional, male world that cultivates confidence, arrogance, and workaholism. The discovery by one of the firm's partners of a KS lesion on Beckett's forehead eventually leads to his illegal dismissal and to his subsequent search for justice, which fuels the film's plot. Yet, though the plot revolves around the injustice Beckett encounters (and though Hanks, not Washington, won the Best Actor Oscar), *Philadelphia* is never really Beckett's story. Instead, his plight is merely a way to depict the transformation of Miller, the straight lawyer who represents Middle America's homophobia. The relationship between Beckett and Miller functions as a metaphor for the relationship between Middle America and gay white men.

Throughout the film, Joe Miller is the mouthpiece for people's fear and hatred of homosexuals. Similar to films on racism in which the focus is on the prejudiced white person's transformation rather than on the African American's life in a racist society, *Philadelphia* tells the story of Joe Miller's education in AIDS awareness and homophobia. This film educates heterosexual Americans on AIDS and gay life through the perspective of a likable, successful, black, heterosexual lawyer. (It is surely no accident that Miller is played by Washington, a star actor who is the black equivalent of Hanks, one of Hollywood's most popular white actors.)

Much of Miller's education is about the myths of AIDS. Just after Beckett tells Miller that he has AIDS, Miller recoils from Beckett's handshake. Miller immediately visits his doctor, who informs him that merely shaking the hand of someone with AIDS cannot infect him. The theme of the film becomes clear at this point: Miller, the "average" American, must become educated about AIDS and gay people. By the film's end and Beckett's death, Miller has changed; he has transformed from hating and fearing gay men to being tolerant of them.

In a further attempt to educate straight people about AIDS, *Philadelphia* utilizes a baby motif for multiple purposes. Graphic depictions of the effects of AIDS on the body are softened with images of newborns. Furthermore, the presence of newborns serves a generic narrative function: where there is death there is life; death and birth are connected, intertwined, fundamental human experiences, and heterosexual reproduction eases the fear and loss.

In one key scene, Beckett holds his sister's new infant. Seated next to him is his lover, Miguel, who watches Beckett cradle the baby, while Beckett's parents, siblings, and the siblings' spouses smile approvingly. The message here is clear: this family loves its gay member, evident in that it allows him access to the vulnerable, innocent baby. When Beckett's sister asks her brother if he wants her to take the baby, he replies that he's fine, and she smiles. This is one of many scenes that teach families in the audience how to be like the Becketts.

Near the end of the first act of the movie, Joe Miller becomes the proud father of a new baby girl. When Beckett shows up at Miller's office to ask him to take his case, Beckett begins the conversation by referring to the congratulation cards and cigars on Miller's desk. Later, Miller witnesses Beckett's harassment at a law library and responds by coming to his aid, thus making his first crisis decision. Once again, Beckett begins their conversation by asking about Miller's new baby. Each scene is meant to challenge the stereotype that gay men are child molesters who can't be trusted with children. Replacing this negative image with the image of white gay men as possessing the same human values of intimacy and family that straight people cherish becomes a main agenda of the film.

What complicates *Philadelphia*'s educational agenda is the film's representation of race. bell hooks argues that Miguel, Beckett's Latino lover, played by Antonio Banderas, "is portrayed as living only to be the little mammy, taking care of the great white man" (*Reel*, 87). hooks finds the relationship between Andrew Beckett and Joe Miller also unbelievable from the standpoint of racism: "Nothing in the script of *Philadelphia* even hints at what would lead Denzel Washington's character to divest himself of his homophobia and take time away from his wife and newborn baby girl to work overtime defending a gay white lawyer with AIDS. The implication is that 'good' white males are inherently worthy, deserving of care, and, of course, always superior to black men in their values and actions, even when they are sick and dying" (*Reel*, 87).

However, even though Joe Miller is a symbol of acceptable, nonthreatening black male subjectivity served up to white audiences, he is allowed to have some degree of agency and a developed personal life. When his daughter is born, he is shown surrounded by family and community; at work, he is the boss and he is successful. Even as the film problematically has him learn the lesson that infringements on gay rights constitute real discrimination that must concern straight people, Joe Miller is more than a foil to Andrew Beckett. Yet in the second Hollywood film on AIDS, the

African American female protagonist, in contrast to Joe Miller, learns a different lesson: submission and self-sacrifice. Similar to *Philadelphia, Boys on the Side* (1995) uses the theme of AIDS to explore race, but its focus is on white popular feminism and relations between white and black women, at black women's expense.

African American Women and Film

The lives of women of color have rarely been the focus of commercial Hollywood films.[7] Elite white male power structures in Hollywood still determine which women's narratives are "valuable"—in terms of profit and social control—and which are not. Predictably, white, heterosexual, middle-class women stand in for elite men's "valuable" property, while working-class women, lesbians, and all women of color are symbolically less valuable or not valued at all.[8]

Until the late 1960s, most black actors were still cast in Hollywood films as happy, childlike dancers, singers, or musicians, or as affable maids and servants who functioned as human props and foils to the white stars. In Shirley Temple movies, for example, the adorable curly-haired girl forged a relationship with her black dance teachers and servants. In Mae West movies, the outrageously sexy star, beloved today by both gay men and feminists, was shown surrounded by adoring black maids who answered to her every whim. Hattie McDaniel's skilled performance as Mammy in *Gone With the Wind* reinforced the notion that, as Donald Bogle puts it, "black shoulders were made to cry on" (153). As with many black female roles, Mammy is not allowed to possess a complex life of her own. Her only means of self-expression is through her influence and care of the suffering yet "difficult" Scarlett O'Hara.[9] The all-too-familiar cultural fantasy of the black woman as "the mighty nurturer" continues to structure the kinds of roles black female actors play in contemporary American films (Bogle, 298). The only two black female actors to win Academy Awards to date are Hattie McDaniel and Whoopi Goldberg, both of whom won in the best supporting actress category for "mammy" roles, another clear indication of the pervasive values of the Hollywood racial patriarchy.[10]

Aside from the controversial film *The Color Purple*, Whoopi Goldberg has been repeatedly cast in films in which she is the sole black character surrounded by an all-white cast. In addition, Goldberg is often presented in an updated version of the mammy/servant role. In *Ghost*, her Oscar-winning role, she plays a wacky medium who is compelled to reunite a grief-stricken white woman with her dead, yuppie husband (Bogle, 329). In *The Long Walk Home*, she plays a domestic servant who "humanizes" her white southern employer, and in *Clara's Heart* she assumes the role of a beautifully dressed, wise, live-in Jamaican maid who nurtures a neglected, rich, white boy. In the 1996 film *Bogus*, Goldberg once again portrays a single woman who, after the sudden death of her best friend, becomes guardian of her late friend's child. As in *Clara's Heart*, the little boy is white and emotionally distraught.

While Goldberg's characters are portrayed as the moral center in these films, and, as in *Clara's Heart*, the character's own personal struggles are slightly developed, her characters are consistently without a separate romantic/personal/communal life of their own. In almost all of her movies, Goldberg is consistently denied an on-screen romance. As Bogle notes, "The very idea of Whoopi Goldberg as a romantic film personality was unacceptable to certain audiences. Filmmakers seemed to view her as an asexual creature from another universe." Unfortunately, Goldberg's role as Jane DeLuca in *Boys on the Side* follows this dominant pattern of the desexualized, updated mammy.[11]

Hailed by *New York Times* film critic Janet Maslin as "one of the strongest Hollywood movies to deal with AIDS thus far," *Boys on the Side* breaks ground as the first commercial film with well-known actors—Whoopi Goldberg, Mary-Louise Parker, and Drew Barrymore—to address the neglected issue of women and AIDS and to present an out, black lesbian character (C3). *Boys* attracted a mixed audience, but it was primarily marketed as a women's/gay film. Lesbians and bisexual women were anxious to see a major star play "gay," while heterosexual women of varied racial and cultural identifications were drawn to the topic of AIDS and to the women's bonding theme made popular by *Thelma and Louise* (1991).

The story begins with Jane DeLuca as an angry, isolated, unsuccessful lead singer for an otherwise all-white, all-male rock band. In the opening scene, Jane is singing a rendition of Janis Joplin's "Piece of My Heart" before an indifferent audience in a seedy New York nightclub. One of the club's intoxicated patrons, a young white woman, is laughing and flirting with her male date and disturbing Jane's concentration. Insulted by this woman's rude behavior, Jane boldly approaches her after the set. The woman immediately assumes that Jane is a waitress who has come to clear away the bottles and glasses. Jane explains that she is the singer in the band and humorously confronts the woman's annoying behavior.

Throughout the first forty minutes of the film, Jane is smart, confrontational, and sarcastic. She swears unflinchingly at a New York City cab driver, wears a black leather jacket, a symbol of "toughness," and is forceful and opinionated. When Jane's co-worker informs her that the band has lost its gig at the club, this seventeen-year veteran of the music club scene swiftly decides to quit the band and move to Los Angeles in search of new work and a new life. She answers an ad for a ride share placed in the newspaper by Robin, played by Mary-Louise Parker, and Jane and Robin meet for lunch.

Robin and Jane are the archetypal odd couple. Whereas Jane is abrasive, tough, and "butch," Robin, a successful real estate agent, is controlled, ultrafeminine—she's often dressed in soft cashmere and angora—and fastidious. With great reluctance (and with no real options), Jane agrees to the ride share with Robin, whom she calls "the whitest woman on the face of the earth."

The movie charts the growth and transformation in Jane and Robin's unlikely friendship as they travel across the country accompanied by Jane's cute but goofy friend Holly, played by Drew Barrymore. Together the three women bond as they confront Holly's experiences with domestic violence, Robin's struggle as a woman with AIDS, and Jane's encounters with racism and homophobia. The film ends with Robin's death from AIDS, the birth of Holly's biracial baby, and Jane in pretty much the same position as when the story started: without a job, a girlfriend, or a viable cultural community.

The Desexualization of Jane

Two film critics, Janet Maslin of the *New York Times* and Elizabeth Pincus of *Gay Community News*, refer to the production of tears in *Boys on the Side*, but neither reviewer considers the impact of this sentimentality on the presentation of Goldberg's Jane.[12] Maslin, in line with the views of academic feminists such as Jane Tompkins, sees the film as presenting a poignant tale of women's solidarity and power.

Indeed, the film is a statement about women bonding, forged in a popular feminist style. Some clear markers of this are the title; the all-women's soundtrack featuring the work of Melissa Etheridge, the Indigo Girls, Annie Lennox, and Bonnie Raitt; Robin's reference to Anne Sexton's "In Celebration of My Uterus"; and occasional nods to *Thelma and Louise*. Yet the bland notion of universality that accompanies these signposts minimizes many experiences and identities while magnifying others. The film conflates sameness with a homogeneous, sentimental universalism, belittling difference, conflict, and contradiction, which are by implication divisive and "unsisterly."

Yet, from Maslin's perspective, *Boys on the Side* is a successful film: "sharp," "funny," and one that "creates an unexpected groundswell of real emotion" (C3). Comparing it to *Thelma and Louise* and *Terms of Endearment*, Maslin celebrates *Boys on the Side* for its ability to "[blur] lines of race and gender with surprising ease" (C3).[13]

But does the film blur the lines of race and gender, or does it deny race in favor of white gender? It is important to point out that blurring lines of race and gender is not the same as acknowledging the power of difference, and this is a distinction that both Maslin and the movie miss. For "blurring" race and gender fails to decenter whiteness—Goldberg's character, despite the "blurring," is still marginalized.

Maslin does note, however, that Jane is "the quintessential outsider as the film begins" and that Goldberg herself is "Hollywood's most uncategorizable star" (C3). Yet this inexplicable outsider status seems irrelevant to Maslin, who declares that *Boys on the Side* has finally provided Goldberg with "a role that suits her talents" (C3).[14]

In a sort of quick afterthought, Maslin does comment on the "small irony" that *Boys on the Side* "depicts [AIDS] in terms of a straight white woman," and on the unfortunate decision to present Jane's sexuality "in terms of metaphor and wisecracking rather than actual physicality" (C3). But for viewers with even the slightest awareness of the politics of AIDS in America, this choice will not be surprising: a white, heterosexual, middle-class woman, even one who contracts HIV as Robin does through a one-night stand with a bartender, is more likely, given racial, class, and sexual politics, to garner visibility than a black or working-class woman who contracts HIV in exactly the same way.

Robin's inevitable death from AIDS takes on broad, heroic meanings; she becomes a symbol of lost youth, unrealized young motherhood, and the impossibility of heterosexual love and marriage. In one scene, Robin can't get HBO in her motel room, so she asks Jane if she can watch *The Way We Were* on the television in hers. Jane joins her in a tearful viewing, during which Robin confesses that she's not "very liberated. . . . I want a husband with a decent job. I want two kids, a boy and a girl, in that order. And a salt-box Colonial with three bedrooms, a sunporch, a stairway with a white banister, and a convertible den." Through her association with Jane, Robin gradually develops a feminist consciousness, but it is one that aggressively includes traditional (white) motherhood, marriage, and monogamy above all else. Robin symbolizes "valuable" womanhood and the American Dream in a way that outsider Jane cannot.

Alongside *Boy*'s vision of women and AIDS are facts such as that black women compose 59 percent of all cases of U.S. women with AIDS, and that in 1993, a study conducted in San Francisco indicated that "HIV seroprevalence was more than three times higher among lesbian and bisexual women than for all women" (Groeger, 4–5). Had she been aware of such facts, perhaps Maslin's discussion of the "small irony" of Robin and the elision of Jane's "actual physicality" would have been more complex.

To Elizabeth Pincus, *Boys on the Side* may be "brash" and "ballsy," with Whoopi Goldberg "bursting onto the screen as a full-blown, not-shy-of-the-'L' word lesbo" (26), but the film's desexualization of Jane disappoints. Pincus angrily argues that Goldberg "is granted a platonic crush on the movie's tragic heterosexual, turning a heretofore bawdy romp into a picture that's maudlin and sterile" (26). Sharing Pincus's frustration were several lesbian viewers who voiced their discontent on an America Online message board: "The lesbian was cynically rendered unlucky-in-love as to make her more palpable for a general audience. Wouldn't the movie have done just as well if Whoopi Goldberg's love life was healthy?"; "In film, lesbians are usually a sexual void"; "My friend said she was sick of seeing Hollywood portray lesbians as 'women who always fall in love with straight women' "; "I am also tired of unrequited lesbian love stories."

These viewers' frustrations with Hollywood's (and society's) inability to allow Jane a love life seem accurate, yet it is revealing that none address the desexualization of Jane in terms of racial politics: the fact that Jane is a black woman surrounded, for the most part, by white people. Pincus, unlike Maslin and the viewers quoted above, questions the film's overly idealized multiracial, intergenerational sisterly solidarity, which she dismisses as "hokey" and "def[ying] belief" (26). But Pincus's discussion of lesbian representation overlooks the historical process of what Wahneema Lubiano refers to as racialized gender. Pincus, like Maslin, does not consider that the black lesbian character, Jane, is stripped of a romantic life not only because of her sexual identity, but also because she is black. Jane is certainly neither celibate by choice nor romantically shut down, as her wistful, sexual-emotional longing for the heterosexual Robin and Holly makes evident. But the fact that she's a black woman also explains her nonexistent love life.

Jane's lack of "actual physicality" exists within the larger historical stereotype of the black woman as innately immoral and hypersexual. As a black lesbian, Jane experiences her sexuality, to borrow from Evelynn Hammonds's theories on black lesbian sexuality, as a "deviant sexuality [that] exists within an already pre-existing deviant sexuality" ("Black," 137). Jane is unconsciously associated with historical narratives of black women's sexuality as excessive, illicit, and taboo.[15]

If we look back at *Boys on the Side* the way the character Blanche White might, we will recognize that the tearful aspect of the film, while potentially moving and empowering to some audiences, may not be experienced as such by many women of color. Homophobia clearly contributes to the desexed, nurturing Jane, but homophobia and racism are inseparable in her characterization, as theoretical work on black women's sexuality makes clear.

Creating the Lesbian Mammy

While audiences and filmmakers may feel uncomfortable with Goldberg playing a heterosexual or homosexual romantic personality, they are, predictably, very much at ease with her in films with a "covert nurturing theme" (Bogle, 331). Patricia Hill Collins explains that "the mammy image is one of an asexual woman, a surrogate mother in blackface devoted to the development of a white family" ("Mammies," 72). Unlike the traditional mammy, Goldberg's mammy role in *Boys on the Side* incorporates her lesbian identity, and her white family consists of two single women under thirty, one of whom has AIDS. Nevertheless, Goldberg's lesbian persona possesses the subordinating traits of the traditional black mammy.

The popularity of the mammy figure originated with the publication of Harriet Beecher Stowe's *Uncle Tom's Cabin* where, as Patricia Turner explains, "Stowe's physical description of Aunt Chole, the faithful wife to Uncle Tom and loyal servant to the Shelby family, set the standard for future fictional representations of mammy figures" (46). Stowe's novel influenced how black women would be imagined in dominant fiction and in visual representations throughout the nineteenth century and provided a legacy that continues to this day. For this reason, Turner argues, *Uncle Tom's Cabin* "is virtually impossible to ignore in a study of race and American popular culture" (67).[16]

The mammy/auntie figure of Stowe's famous novel reappeared in nineteenth-century theatrical adaptations of *Uncle Tom's Cabin,* and in the twentieth century in films and in material culture—salt and pepper shakers, cookie jars, napkin holders, and in almost any object associated with the kitchen. Turner has found that

> Mammy/auntie figures constitute the most frequently depicted character. . . . Draped in calico from head to toe, Aunt Jemima and her cronies pose no sexual threat to their white mistresses. They want to nourish rather than seduce white men. The artifacts they grace belong almost exclusively to the kitchen. . . . The mammy figures convey the notion that genuine fulfillment for black women comes not from raising their own children or feeding their own man (black [heterosexual] families are rarely featured) but from serving in a white family's kitchen. (25)

The film industry's transformation of black women into symbols of benevolence and self-sacrifice is fully evidenced in the mammy character of Jane. Jane nourishes and comforts Robin and Holly through each individual life crisis. She is the rock, the all-giving mother who never asks for nourishment, so devoted is she to these two characters' needs. Jane is stripped of emotional needs in addition to sensuality and desire, for she is an emblem of selfless, sentimental nurturance. The film's refusal to give Jane an interior life of her own, one composed of desires, rage, dreams, memories, pleasure, fears, as well as a visible community, makes this clear. The only role available to her is as a devoted, celibate, lesbian friend/ mammy and second-class citizen. Jane is repeatedly depicted as comforting and emotionally attentive to her adopted white family, yet she is rarely the recipient of their tenderness and care. And while it is true that Goldberg plays Jane as an opinionated, forceful woman, Jane's forcefulness is often in response to these two women and their predicaments. On the whole, Jane's own needs are pushed aside and never articulated.

Jane's initial preoccupation with finding work in Los Angeles as a musician and with healing her own broken heart evaporates as she is pulled into the dilemmas of Robin's and Jane's circumstances. Shortly after their dramatic and narrow escape from Holly's brutish and violent boyfriend, Holly begins to have second thoughts about leaving him and considers returning to this drug-addicted, physically abusive man. Even though Jane is appalled by Holly's decision to return to Nick, she stays by her side and watches Holly cry. Frustrated, Jane walks into the bathroom to enlist Robin's help only to find Robin collapsing onto the cold floor. Jane's attention shifts from Holly to Robin, who is immediately rushed to the hospital in an ambulance. The next scene depicts the exhausted and worried Jane sitting in a hospital waiting room, the sweet little Holly sleeping in her lap, as the doctor informs Jane that Robin has AIDS. In the following scene, Jane is shown comforting Robin as she cries and pulls at the tubes in her nose and arms.

Jane's friendship with these women would not be so stifling if the screenplay gave her other friends and a chosen community; instead Jane has been plunged into the drama of these women's lives unwittingly. But it is what she does with this situation that is disturbing: she inexplicably abandons her former plan to start over in L.A. in order to help Robin and Holly. Three months later, the women are living together in a beautiful house in Tucson, Arizona, and Jane has hooked into a lesbian bar community, but she is still focused on Robin's needs, in terms of both romance and health. In addition to experiencing constant stress and anxiety associated with Robin's AIDS diagnosis, Jane sees her idealized friendship with Robin deteriorate because of misunderstandings about Jane's "crush" on the heterosexual Robin. Meanwhile, the pregnant Holly becomes involved with an idealistic, naive, conservative cop named Abe Lincoln who turns Holly over to the authorities once he learns that she may have been involved in the murder of her battering boyfriend, Nick. Janet Maslin refers to this part of the plot and the courtroom sequence that follows as clumsy and "contrived." But the courtroom drama allows Jane to come out as "gay" in response to an arrogant, feminist-bashing, homophobic prosecutor, and it provides Robin with the opportunity to present her ideas on feminism as sisterly solidarity before she dies.

Significantly, when Robin shows up to testify on Holly's behalf, she says to her estranged friend, Jane, "You are my family and I love you." Jane responds by bending over and picking up Robin's luggage.[17]

In *Boys on the Side*, it is a black, unattractively dressed, desexualized lesbian who, in taking care of a slender, white, middle-class woman with AIDS, serves as a nonthreatening moral compass and role model to an AIDS-phobic audience and society. Similar to Harriet Beecher Stowe's Topsy, Jane is a mischievous entertainer who, through her contact with the more delicate and dying Robin, transforms into a lesbian mammy/caretaker.

Black Women, AIDS, and Silence

Blanche White's analysis of "Mammy-save-me eyes" provides us with a sense of how Neely's character might respond to the relationship between Jane and Robin in *Boys on the Side;* it also uncovers a key mechanism in the production of silence about black women and AIDS in American culture at large. *Boys* obscures its problematic assumptions about race and gender behind the cloak of breaking silence.[18] As Evelynn Hammonds argues, "visibility in and of itself does not erase a history of silence nor does it challenge the structure of power and domination, symbolic and material, that determines what can and cannot be seen" ("Black," 141).[19] A black lesbian character is the ostensible protagonist in *Boys on the Side*, but in fact she is a subtle, contemporary reworking of the good mammy figure who is isolated from communities of color and denied a sexual/romantic relationship. The complex experiences of black women are silenced in this spectacle of a supposedly neutral and "natural" feminist emotionality, complete with an updated beloved black servant figure and a feisty, dying, white heroine.[20] As bell hooks points out, "The racial politics of Hollywood are such that there can be no serious representations of death and dying when the characters are African Americans. Sorrowful black death is not a hot ticket" (*Reel*, 35).

Another puzzling contradiction arises in this "feminist" film when Robin's demise from AIDS is juxtaposed with the antics of Holly, a sexually active childlike woman who seems to have never heard of safer sex or contraceptives—she's eight weeks pregnant when the film opens and won't consider abortion because "it's murder." Maslin describes Holly as possessing the luscious flirtiness of a 1940s pinup girl, but Holly's position in this film is a bit more ideological. The film ends with Holly married to a conservative white cop who, miraculously, accepts her biracial baby. The plight of Robin suggests that yes, even white, heterosexual, educated, "valuable" women contract HIV and develop AIDS; but this message is undermined by the experiences of Holly, who has more unsafe sex than any other character in the entire film and never once considers HIV as an issue—even though her symptomatic housemate contracted HIV through a one-night stand.

On one level, Holly can be read as comic relief from the "heavy" issues so that the movie itself can have a sexy and fun side. But the underlying effect is that pleasure and danger are split off—as are race, class, gender, and sexuality—as if they existed in separate universes, a binary that Carol S. Vance says stems from cultural tradition: "It is all too easy to cast sexual experience as either wholly pleasurable or dangerous; our culture encourages us to do so" (5). It is as if the decision to break silence on women and AIDS is so fraught with anxiety that the narrative makes up for its own bravery by mitigating its message of risk. But breaking silence and creating visibility are not enough to challenge cultural assumptions.

Touched by an Angel

Boys on the Side offers a vision of AIDS and women that hinges on the cliché of the suffering white woman and the black mammy who cares for her. But such an interpretation of the film does not rule out alternative readings. In *"The Color Purple:* Black Women as Cultural Readers," Jacqueline Bobo discusses how black women spectators "filter out that which is negative and select from the work elements [they] can relate to" when presented with the exotic primitive stereotype of African Americans in film and in other forms of popular culture (262). While one cannot rely on this individualistic filtering paradigm to adequately represent or advocate for women in the age of AIDS (nor, as bell hooks suggests in *Reel to Real: Race, Sex, and Class at the Movies*, does such a transgressive filtering process necessarily undermine white supremacist assumptions), it is crucial to analyze spectators' readings of commercial popular culture. For example, Patrice Clark Koelsch argues:

> What may be interpreted as a narrative of erasure or omission for some can be genuinely instructive for another. I remember fuming that *Tootsie* was about a man teaching a woman how to be a woman, while my mother said it really made her think about gender roles. Even now the people with AIDS I work with are usually glad to see themselves "mainstreamed" on television. *Touched by an Angel* is a favorite series. (20)[21]

Similarly, the admittedly problematic emotionality of *Boys on the Side*, coupled with its standard view of death as a "crossing over" or "homecoming," could easily be appropriated by people with or affected by AIDS to articulate self-definition, agency, and resistance.[22] The qualities of emotionality and death as "crossing over" suggest an important dimension of the personal experience of HIV illness, one that biomedical constructions, right-wing moralizing, and political activist renderings have often failed to convey.

As I discussed in Chapter 2, Harriet Beecher Stowe's Little Eva was known as "more angel than ordinary," and when she "crossed over" it was felt that her spirit had never really belonged to the earth. So, too, we encounter a child's innate otherworldliness and angel-like qualities in *Boys on the Side*. During Robin's last hospital stay, shortly before she dies, her deceased baby brother, Tommy, visits her. He is on the other side of her hospital room window, staring and waving. Parker plays this scene skillfully, with just the right mixture of fear, intrigue, disbelief, and desire. The effect is moving and especially comforting to viewers whose lives have been torn apart by AIDS, cancer, or other deaths. The scene provides a consoling vision, one that diffuses the extreme fear and anxiety of death.

Likewise, the choreographer David Rousseve uses images of death as "crossing over" in his AIDS dance theater piece, *The Whispers of Angels*. Rousseve presents visitations with departing spirits as an imaginative way to offer solace and comfort to his beleaguered audience, similar to Stowe's lavish deathbed scenes in *Uncle Tom's Cabin* and to the supernatural communion between the dying Robin and her dead little brother in *Boys on the Side*.[23] Rousseve centers his piece on human beings making the transition from life to death because in his own life as a black gay man he is deeply involved in this process. In addition to a chorus, the choreographer includes several dancing angels, many of whom are people who have died of AIDS. "Angels help with the idea of losing people, of people crossing over," Rousseve has explained. "The concept soothes me: death is a continuum with life. Angels are a source of comfort, an unabashedly spiritual thing" (Zimmer, 63).

In the dance, Rousseve plays a black gay man dying of AIDS who, just as he dies, is miraculously reunited with his estranged father. The idea of the continuum between life and death that makes death a "crossing over"; the highly emotional reconciliation between the dying gay man and his estranged, dead father; the belief that when we die we become angels—these are all stock images and ideas found in sentimental aesthetic practice. Yet Rousseve deepens his use of these traditions when he explains that the hopeful notions of death as a "crossing over" and as a productive homecoming are fundamental ideas of the black church.

Similarly, Lynn Wardley has argued that notions of transcendence and spirituality found in nineteenth-century American sentimental writing unwittingly possess a complex "infusion" of West African spirituality. Both Wardley and Rousseve offer a view of sentimental transcendence while also challenging its association with a Eurocentric view. The belief that death is a glorious, long-awaited homecoming and that objects and places possess a spiritual animation is not naturally or inevitably Christian, white, middle-class, or Euro-American.

At the same time, Rousseve, unlike Wardley, points out that "crossing over" and becoming an angel must not act as a "tranquilizer" for the audience. Existence may, in fact, be better once we have "crossed over," but that promise must not interfere with the business of helping people who struggle in their bodily lives.[24] Ultimately, Rousseve agrees with a skeptical critic who says that "it doesn't help us in the here and now to say you're going to be an angel" (Zimmer, 63).

It is highly unusual to find such a nuanced, complex view of sentimentality in a work on AIDS, a view that does not use emotional intensity or sentimental transcendence as spectacle to drown out the material, political, social, and economic context of the pandemic. Rousseve explains that the use of angels in his piece is a "paradox," and that he himself holds a conflicted view of sentimental spirituality. From this imaginative perspective, death does have some meaning as it ushers us into a better place where we can still communicate with those who have left us and with those whom we have left. Yet, at the same time, Rousseve maintains a skepticism about the very view that he cherishes and lavishly displays in his dance. "The black church," he explains, "has been criticized, rightfully, for being tranquilizing. . . . That's the paradox of the piece: people cross over, they're still with us, but things are still screwed up. They're dying all around us" (Zimmer, 63).

With this last comment, Rousseve offers a contradictory view of his own artistic practice, a complexity that *Boys on the Side,* and much work on AIDS, lack. He openly considers how concepts such as "crossing over" and reunion with departed spirits can and do distract us from the problems of the living. Yet the transformative potential of both Rousseve's construction of AIDS and that of *Boys on the Side* is obvious to anyone who has been made to feel invisible by either abstract intellectualization or medicalized discourse. Taken together, both texts highlight "the moral efficacy of sympathy" as a fundamental issue of AIDS criticism (Schilling, 110).

Ann Cvetkovich specifically argues for a balance between free, emotional expression/mourning and political action in response to AIDS, not an eradication of emotional expression. I believe it is unwise to dismiss the moving vision of Rousseve's dance piece or to discount entirely the problematic gesture of sisterly solidarity in *Boys on the Side.* It is not the representation of emotion per se that is at issue; it is the way in which representations of emotional suffering are often used to conceal other complexities, experiences, and social realities. In fact, like Douglas Crimp in his 1989 essay "Mourning and Militancy," Cvetkovich warns against an approach to AIDS that would deny the full expression of emotion:

> The most effective activism might require both mourning *and* militancy, the recognition both of what can be changed because AIDS is not simply a biological problem but a social one, and of what cannot be changed in the face of death. The repression of mourning because of the need to confront without sentimentality how sexism, racism, and homophobia structure the

incidence and treatment of AIDS might constitute a dangerous avoidance of the reality of suffering, an avoidance that creates not just individual psychic distress but political difficulties. The expression of feeling and activism need not be at odds, although they often are when affect is represented or experienced as natural or inevitable. (127)

The problem lies not in human emotion itself, but in the trivialization of human emotion and in passing off suffering and emotional expression as an ahistorical, "natural" activity.[25] Yet the complex inspiration and solace that aspects of the film provide—in particular, the spiritual notion of death as crossover—must be acknowledged. Rousseve's use of the "crossing over" theme and Robin's visitations from her baby brother turned angel point to some of these moments.

In addition, *Boys on the Side* does succeed in breaking the resounding silence on women and AIDS in mainstream film, as do Maslin's and Pincus's film reviews. In contrast, *Philadelphia* includes a woman character in only a minor, incidental part, which is a more prevalent construction of women in AIDS discourse, even when women themselves are HIV infected. *Boys* eschews this marginal positioning of women in the pandemic by giving the central role to a woman character who falls outside the ideological "risk group" fabrication. We watch her swallow her AZT, struggle with nausea, and prepare for death. Again, for audience viewers who have personal or political experience with HIV/AIDS in women, the story is powerful.

Robin's deep human fear of mortality and physical pain; her intense feelings of social isolation; her desperate need for her mother; her longing for romantic and sexual love; the painful and vivid memories of the loss of her six-year-old brother to cancer; and Jane's overall reaction to Robin, which suggests that Robin is not the first friend Jane has lost to AIDS, are all representational issues with which many viewers will be familiar.

The Education of Jane

Despite its breaking ground on AIDS and despite its emotional power, *Boys on the Side* unwittingly promotes a racial hierarchy for women and AIDS which it tries to hide by evoking a watered-down, nostalgic notion of universal feminist solidarity. This is why the Little Eva-like Robin is "touched by an angel" while Jane, similar to Stowe's Topsy, is not. In effect, in addressing the enormously painful issue of women and AIDS, the film presents a hopeful, humane vision of caretaking yet reinforces the paradigm of women as inevitable, "natural" caregivers and insidiously constructs black women as comic maids and sentimentalized mammies. Furthermore, Robin's characterization also hinges on the unacknowledged agenda and interests of privileged heterosexual males who demand this type of female character as male property and dupe. This, after all, is the hidden subtext of many AIDS narratives; however, being socially constructed as a "valuable" woman by elite men is not the same as having social, economic, and legal equality.

On the whole, Whoopi Goldberg's Jane (unlike Barbara Neely's Blanche) loses her critical ability to resist the dominating effects of white sentimental corporate power. Goldberg's Jane initially feels put off by Robin's white-bread physical appearance, her adoration of Carole King and the Carpenters, and her penchant for women's romantic "weepies," such as *The Way We Were* and *An Officer and a Gentleman*—examples of white romantic culture that Robin cherishes and that Jane finds incomprehensible and offensive. But before too long, Jane is humming, and even singing and playing, Carpenters' songs. Viewers are asked to celebrate Jane and Robin's racial reconciliation, which symbolizes that these two otherwise incompatible women/cultures have forged a bond despite insurmountable odds. However, the burden of change and compromise falls on Jane. Since Jane barely has a world of her own, the more she becomes immersed in the world of Robin, the less she seems like the independent, East Village musician we meet when the movie opens.

Following in the mammy tradition, Jane does emerge as an influence on the white heroine, when Robin admits in front of an entire courtroom that she's not gay but "at times I understand the inclination." In another instance, Jane's "influence" is more problematic. In one of the film's many intertextual references, Jane directly evokes *Gone With the Wind*'s Mammy and Scarlett, although with a twist.[26] Here, Jane is "humorously" constructed as the hypersexual black woman while comically parodying the figure of the sentimentalized mammy. She persuades the prudish, uptight Robin to utter the word *cunt*, liberating Robin from her nice, sexually repressed, white girl training—"You free, Miz' Scarlett, you free!" Yet it is impossible not to read this scene as representing the black woman as stand-in for the "good" white woman's repressed sexuality.[27]

Ultimately, *Boys on the Side* is a classic Hollywood education plot. By the movie's end, Jane changes from a wisecracking skeptic to a caretaking desexualized "sister." The inciting incident that leads Jane down a different path and alters her life forever occurs when she quits the band and agrees to drive across the country with Robin and Holly. Jane, the protagonist of this education plot, learns how to be less gruff and more tender, and that racism and homophobia are her problem; if only Jane weren't so angry and sarcastic, the film suggests, then she would be a happier woman. The film's underlying project is "working out" the initial racial-sexual-cultural tension through a racial patriarchy conveyed by sentimental feminism.

In the next chapter I will examine three contemporary novels by and about black women and HIV/AIDS, and will explore how each novel draws from black feminist literary traditions to dismantle the racial and gender silences on black women, girls, and HIV/AIDS, and yet how each utilizes visions of gendered caretaking.

CHAPTER 5

WHAT LOOKS LIKE PROGRESS

BLACK FEMINIST NARRATIVES ON HIV/AIDS

> Most folks continue to articulate a vision of racial uplift
> that prioritizes the needs of males and valorizes con-
> ventional notions of gender roles.
>
> bell hooks, "Ain't She Still a Woman?"

Since the release of *Boys on the Side,* progressive black feminist discourse on HIV has emerged on the literary scene. Charlotte Watson Sherman's *touch,* Sapphire's *Push,* and Pearl Cleage's *What Looks Like Crazy on an
Ordinary Day* forge a dramatic convergence between evolving commentary
on women and AIDS and black women's writing, and for this alone these
three texts are worthy of critical attention. They are trailblazers in the way
they draw on black feminist literary innovations to imagine the story of
AIDS from black women's standpoints. All three novels focus on HIV in
black women and girls, and all challenge the still standard assumption that
AIDS is a disease of the socially unacceptable and guilty. They also candidly and repeatedly challenge the black community's silences on HIV.

At the same time that they address (and protest) racial and gender silence on the epidemic, each novel utilizes traditional conceptions of femininity, particularly in terms of gender and caretaking. African American
women's mothering, caretaking, and community activism are often expressions of political and cultural self-preservation rather than instances
of diminishment and destructive self-denial—these latter themes are often
associated with white middle-class women's experiences of mothering.[1]
Mothering for African American women can be a radical, resistant act, one
that slaveholders attempted to deny them—yet women still mothered—
and one that continues to be threatened by economic racism and racial vi-

olence. But mothering for African American women can also be an experience of self-obliteration, a view Nella Larsen vividly dramatized in her award-winning novel, *Quicksand*. *Quicksand* ends with Helga Crane, who has been paralyzed by depression, regaining enough physical and emotional strength to get out of bed only to realize that she is pregnant with her fifth child. Marriage and motherhood, when not freely chosen, are a prison from which Helga can escape only through death or submission.

In the context of AIDS, interpreting the needs of children and community as synonymous with women's needs and health supports the very ideology that puts women's bodies at risk in the first place. The fact that women can physically give birth to and nurse children, and men cannot, is a biological difference that is still used to justify certain kinds of ideology, such as that nurturing, sacrifice, and selflessness are women's authentic work.[2] Women who do not give birth to children, who are not literal mothers, are still expected to act as metaphoric mothers, a construction that preserves the link between woman and care as an act of nature.[3] These three novels by Sherman, Sapphire, and Cleage actively address AIDS from a black feminist literary perspective, but they also subtly grapple with, and in some instances reinscribe, the figure of the nurturing woman as the key to stability and compassion in the age of epidemic.

Such an interpretation of these novels is not rooted in an exegesis of these writers' supposed flaws—political or aesthetic. Instead, I argue that the novels are part of a larger social and historical pattern that sanctifies the narrative of mythic womanhood by evoking the inevitability of female self-sacrifice. As bell hooks points out with regard to contemporary film, a text can "have incredibly revolutionary standpoints merged with conservative ones" (*Reel*, 3). Revolutionary and conservative standpoints in print and visual culture on AIDS and the role played by sentimental ideas of women's sacrifice in the conveyance of these standpoints are the subject of this book, but nowhere are revolutionary and conservative perspectives more dramatically merged and conflicted than in these three novels. Traditional conceptions of care and sacrifice compete with forceful, creative black feminist narratives on women, gender, sexuality, and HIV.

Henry Louis Gates observes that "the tensions that beset any project of emancipation . . . illustrat[e] the difficulties of ever escaping entirely the confines of patriarchal discourse" (15). All three of these novels seek to emancipate readers from the most conspicuous racial and gender stereotypes and assumptions common in HIV discourse. But given that they take on the subject of women and HIV, a topic that threatens and bolsters patriarchal power, it is not surprising that conceptions of gender and caretaking emerge in each book, suggesting once again that gendered ideas of women's innate caretaking are integral to AIDS narratives. Even in narratives that actively resist the confines of white supremacy and patriarchy, and even in narratives that rely on African American women's political conceptions of nurturance and sacrifice, feminine sacrifice emerges as an unspoken ideal. I interpret these contradictions and tensions as opportunities to argue that race, gender, and care are inextricably connected in the discourse of AIDS.

Each novel offers a unique signpost indicating the extent to which representations of the pandemic rely on the image of sacrificial woman for their own intelligibility. Sherman's, Sapphire's, and Cleage's books not only tell stories about black women and AIDS; they expose the *centrality* of women, sacrifice, and nurturing to cultural conceptions of AIDS. They indicate how entrenched is the symbol of Mother / Woman, and, in the case of *What Looks Like Crazy on an Ordinary Day*, present an alternative model of sacrifice and care. Before I turn to an analysis of how *touch, Push,* and *What Looks Like Crazy* offer forceful black feminist narratives on HIV at the same time that they nourish gendered conceptions of care and sacrifice, I want to focus on the history informing the revolutionary aspects of these books.

Betrayers or Defenders

Until recently, few literary texts authored by African Americans addressed HIV in black women. Homophobia, racism, and sexism in publishing, education, medicine, and the family are clearly some of the fundamental reasons for this absence, but a complex reticence about HIV in black communities has also contributed to the denial of women and AIDS (Boykin; Hammonds, "Race"; Schoofs, "Black Up"). According to Mario Cooper, co-director of the 1996 Harvard AIDS Institute conference on AIDS in African Americans, "except possibly for slavery, nothing in our history will have killed so many black people in such a short time as AIDS" (quoted in Schoofs, "Black Up," 45). Most African Americans, like most

Americans, do not interpret the epidemic as equivalent to slavery or as a predicament worthy of a full-scale civil rights mobilization. Yet recent Centers for Disease Control statistics reveal that HIV/AIDS is a central experience in African American communities. Twice as many young black men die of AIDS as die of homicide; one out of three black men between the ages of 25 and 44 has died of AIDS; and one out of five black women in this same age group has died (Schoofs, "Black Up," 45). Furthermore, the Harvard AIDS Institute predicts that early in the new century more than half of all AIDS cases in the United States will be African Americans.[4]

At the same time, euphoric news accounts of cutting-edge combination drug therapies have led many to believe that the epidemic is over in the United States. The fact that many individuals cannot tolerate the intricate new combination drug regimes, or that most who need these treatments often lack the financial wherewithal and health insurance to access them, is repeatedly ignored (Schoofs, "Black Up," 45; Shernoff, 16). For many poor people, the so-called end of AIDS is one more example of how the story of the epidemic is constructed so that people of color and women are virtually erased. For example, while the overall number of deaths from AIDS among white men dropped in 1996, a 3 percent increase in women's deaths from AIDS occurred in the same period (Denison, "AIDS Deaths," 4).

These were some of the issues discussed at the Harvard AIDS Institute conference, which attracted the participation of many prominent leaders, and was co-organized by Henry Louis Gates Jr., director of African American studies at Harvard. The purpose of the professional gathering was to confront the devastating toll that AIDS is taking on African Americans. Much discussion centered on the startling fact that although African Americans compose just 12 percent of America's population, they make up "40 per cent of all AIDS cases, more than half the female cases, and more than 60 per cent of children with AIDS" (Schoofs, "Black Up," 45).

Homophobia and the stigma of drug addiction were cited as key causes of apathy and denial (Schoofs, "Black Up," 45).[5] For example, though the conference coordinators invited members of the Congressional Black Caucus, the executive director of the NAACP, and the president of the National Urban League, not one member or representative from these organizations attended (Schoofs, "Black Up," 45). The failure of many prominent black church leaders to attend may suggest a profound level of fear and denial. There are indications that serious organizing on the impact of

HIV in black communities is occurring.[6] Some black church, political, and health leaders who have lost family, friends, and community members to the disease are addressing HIV, but the silences on HIV within diverse black communities, as in most communities, is still very real.[7]

Contemporary silences on HIV in black communities have extremely complex causes and meanings. Historically, black leaders and social reformers have used reticence on issues concerning sexuality as a strategic defense against racism. As Keith Cylar explains, "To counter white bigotry. . . . African Americans often try to present a flawless image. Anyone who deviates from that ideal—such as those who are at highest risk for HIV—face extra ostracism for 'betraying the race.' Then there is the widespread fear that if the truth about who is getting AIDS is known, whites will use it as another club to pummel blacks" (quoted in Schoofs, "Black Up," 45). The more that black communities feel besieged by an illness that is associated with white gay men and illegal drug use, the more these same black communities adopt a protective silence. Denial within black communities on AIDS and issues of sexuality differs, in a few crucial areas, from the denial and responses of mainstream (and nonmainstream) white America.

Evelynn Hammonds has been analyzing responses to HIV in black communities since 1987. Her theories confirm Cylar's view that contemporary silence on AIDS is related to the taboo subjects of sexuality, homosexuality, and drug use. Thus, by not talking about or addressing AIDS directly, some black communities feel that they are "defending" their communities and "race" from the historically entrenched stereotypes that the epidemic engenders. A sexually conservative rhetoric may or may not reflect what black communities actually practice, but as a political strategy, it acts as a bulwark against white bigotry.

Racialized Sexualities

The legacy of "defending one's name" continues to influence how contemporary black women speak and write about their sexuality, bodies, and lives. AIDS evokes old racist stereotypes of black women as innately promiscuous and diseased (Hammonds, "Missing," "Black"). In discussing these stereotypes of African American women, Hammonds repeatedly uses the concept "racialized sexuality," which is the "powerful effect that race has on the construction and representation of gender and sexuality" ("Black," 130). Racialized sexualities are central to conceptions of HIV, as contemporary media reports indicate.

Black women's resistance to racist representations of their sexuality has an extensive history in the United States. In "Jezebel and Mammy: The Mythology of Female Slavery," Deborah Gray White outlines the historical origins of sexual myths of black women (*Aren't,* 26–61). The fantasy of the wanton black female temptress was created by white men and women as a rationalization of the repeated mass rapes of black women by white men during and after slavery. It is a conception of black female sexuality that has caused, and continues to cause, enormous pain, distortion, and violence. In more recent research, White and other scholars address how educated black women responded to these prevailing sexualized, racialized narratives and stereotypes (D. G. White, "Private," 103–23). Since at least the late nineteenth century, African American women club leaders, churchwomen, writers, and activists have wrestled with several stereotypes, especially that of the hypersexual black woman. Many African American women dealt—and deal—with this hypersexual image by adopting a sexually conservative rhetoric as a political strategy (Davis, 19).

The black women's club movement of the late nineteenth and early twentieth centuries encouraged women to "defend" their race against the relentless accusation that all black women were immoral. Some black women were encouraged by middle-class leaders to devote their lives to "racial uplift" and to the creation of respectable heterosexual families, regardless of their actual desires and social realities. Other black women willingly assumed a desexualized self-presentation as a psychological coping mechanism against violent white supremacy. In either case, white supremacy meant that black women's right to self-definition was greatly hindered.

It was not uncommon for middle-class black women of the club movement to judge other women unfit—in particular, working-class women and sex workers—when their sexuality and self-presentations did not conform to a supermoral image. Many black clubwomen saw the "improvement" of black women as their political mission, and they often resented and were intolerant of women who were different.[8] Thus, the work of

countering repeated charges of sexual immorality and impropriety became intertwined with black women's desexualization.

The legacy of "defending one's name" continues to influence how contemporary black women speak and write about their sexuality, bodies,
and lives. AIDS has revived all the familiar scapegoat discourses, bigoted
ideas of gender, and the unresolved anxieties about black women's sexuality and sexual diversity in a racist country. Sapphire's answer to the
problem of silences on sexuality and AIDS is direct and to the point: "We
have to stop thinking that talking about the problem is causing the problem. The problem exists. The question is what are we going to do about it"
(quoted in Bailey).

Black Feminist Literary Traditions and AIDS

Black women writers' literary traditions have paved the way for Sherman's, Sapphire's, and Cleage's fictional accounts of HIV/AIDS in girls
and women. Despite the code of silence on sexuality, many black women
writers have boldly addressed issues associated with sexuality and gender
in their texts for decades, creating literary traditions that address numerous controversial and difficult themes. Domestic violence, incest, infanti-
cide, matricide, internalized racism, intraracial discrimination, passing,
sexual harassment, female genital mutilation, lesbian relationships, slavery, rape, cancer, abortion, tuberculosis, poverty, interracial relationships,
biracial identities, and male homosexuality are some of the themes dramatized in black women's literature stemming back, in some cases, to the
nineteenth century. Black women writers have long rejected aspects of the
"defenders or betrayers" binary, as evident in the work of Nella Larsen,
Zora Neale Hurston, Toni Morrison, Ann Petry, Audre Lorde, Alice
Walker, Gloria Naylor, and Barbara Smith, to name just a few. These writers evade the moralist legacy of the black women's club and church-based
movements while always honoring them for their social activism. Likewise, many of these writers reject the desexualization of black women,
even as a defense against racism.

Hurston's focus on the theme of women's struggle for self-defined individuality in the character of Janie Crawford is such an example (Gates, 15).
Morrison's Sethe, traumatized by slavery, racism, thwarted creativity, and

her inability to practice a self-affirming motherhood, resorts to "unwomanly" violence. Walker's Celie restores her battered self through the sexual love of another black woman. Lorde's landmark essay, "Uses of the Erotic," candidly celebrates black lesbian sexuality and has influenced generations of diverse women writers and activists, as have her essays and poetry on interracial love, African lesbian traditions, medical racism, and the politics of breast cancer. Shame, secrecy, and self-imposed invisibility around issues of race, gender, history, health, and sexuality are countered with healing images, explosive emotion, sexual self-esteem, and personal power. Despite these courageous thematic traditions and the stunning literary techniques that accompany them, only a few contemporary women writers explore black women's individualities, sexuality, and histories in relation to HIV/AIDS.

As a result, *touch*, *Push*, and *What Looks Like Crazy* emerge as watershed moments, strategic responses both to the silences within African American cultures on HIV and to the predominant racist and gendered ideologies of AIDS used to construct black women. In 1993, Charlotte Watson Sherman was one of the first to initiate a black feminist literary intervention with the publication of her anthology, *Sisterfire: Black Womanist Fiction and Poetry.* Under a section heading, "Prelude to an Endnote: The Body's Health," Sherman included an interesting array of poetry and short fiction on HIV, including an excerpt from what would become her novel *touch*. In 1995, Sherman continued to fill the vacuum with the publication of *touch*, one of the first narratives on HIV from the standpoint of a black heterosexual woman character.

In June 1996, Sapphire's controversial novel *Push* appeared, and in 1997 Pearl Cleage's *What Looks Like Crazy on an Ordinary Day* was published, offering another clear signal of an evolving black feminist literary discourse on the epidemic.[9] Both Sherman's and Sapphire's novels, as their titles suggest, focus on bodies. These "physical" titles highlight women's and girls' bodies as sites of power and ingenuity as well as of oppression and pain. All three books are organized around black female protagonists who are HIV positive yet engaged in self-determination and creative self-exploration, and all three novels adopt a diary/epistolary format.[10]

Alice Walker used the epistolary format to augment the perspective of Celie, an overlooked, overworked, and marginalized girl, and, similarly, each of these writers experiments with the diary and epistolary genre in order to give their women characters a privileged position in the text. Sherman intersperses third-person narration with the protagonist's journal entries as a way to stress the character's highly developed identity as an artist as well as her emotional devastation when she tests HIV positive. With the most direct nod to Walker, Sapphire opens *Push* with a dramatic line about incest, "I was left back when I was twelve because I had a baby for my fahver," and then uses the girl's subsequent entries to record her transformation into a young poet and mother. Cleage also employs the journal form to address explosive, taboo themes, such as the violence of traditional black male heterosexual dominance and the hypocrisy of conservative black Christianity.[11] Each novel adapts the diary and letter form as a way to reject the constraints and repression of the dominant culture, but also to protest the oppression black women experience by their own communities.

From Artist to Teacher

In Sherman's *touch*, Rayna Sargent is an introspective, unconventional, thirty-four-year-old middle-class artist who makes her living as a hot-line crisis counselor at a hospital by day and paints at night and on weekends. Before Rayna learns she is HIV positive, she has spent years rejecting her family's and community's expectations of marriage and law school so that she could spend her time developing her work. Her abstract expressionist paintings characteristically convey meaning and feeling through figures of women's bodies and faces and through the use of color. Rayna paints from her dreams and memories and turns to her personal journal for ideas and themes. After she tests positive, she uses the new uncertainty about her body to create: "She had been having a strong urge to paint something new, an image she saw in her mind's eye that was different from anything she had ever done before" (143). Given the dominant image of women in AIDS discourse as emblems of chaos, self-sacrifice, or victimhood, Rayna's struggle to maintain an artist's identity, despite testing positive, is powerful. Rayna's personality is initially forged, not in terms of her relationships, but in terms of her autonomous act of creating art. Rayna's personal journal writing captures her independent and determined spirit, personal qualities that serve her well as a black female artist in a commodity-driven culture: "No one has any power in these pages but me" (203).

In chronicling the multiple effects of the epidemic on her protagonist's life, Sherman bravely addresses several issues that are rarely discussed in literary responses to HIV: sterilization abuse; coercive abortions; refusal of abortion services; black women's AIDS activism; safer sex; heterosexual and homosexual crossings and social alliances; black women's sexual desires; AIDS-phobia in black communities; and gender issues in medical research and treatment. For example, when Rayna investigates how she might enroll in a clinical drug trial, she finds that "most are focused on men. If you have a uterus, they don't want you. They're too afraid of what a drug might do to the unborn child, even if you swear you don't have any plans to have children" (183).

Sherman explores the theme of homophobia in black communities in the character of Novel Lewis, an AIDS-phobic, middle-class psychotherapist who is Rayna's best friend. Rayna begs Novel to collaborate with her on a ceramic tile collage for an art show at Bailey-Boushay House, a residential facility for people with AIDS. Novel says that having her work displayed in an AIDS hospital is too distressing and bad publicity—"What if people think I've got AIDS ?" (6). Sherman also looks at AIDS-phobia through the perspective of Rayna's adoptive parents, Circe and Carr. When Rayna finally tells her parents that she has tested positive, her father wonders "how his Rayna could get something he heard that mostly pretty boys, junkies, and prostitutes got" (135–37).

touch challenges denial on black women and AIDS by creating a middle-class female artist who contracts HIV and confronts her own and her family's and community's hackneyed ideas and silences. But an additional theme runs through the narrative: Rayna's changing view of herself as an artist. Rayna expresses devotion to her art, despite disappointments and obscurity, but once she enters the world of AIDS through friends and through testing positive, she begins to feel ambivalent about maintaining her artistic identity in a world filled with suffering. By the end of the novel, Rayna confesses, "My art is important to me but not more important than the people I care about" (213).

Through Rayna, Sherman seems to be exploring the inhumanity of the Western image of the artist, one based on the white male genius separated from everyday society, a paradigm brilliantly exposed as untenable and deformed—especially for women—in June Jordan's "Waking Up in the Middle of Some American Dreams." Jordan's essay tells the story of a time in her life when she lived completely alone on a desolate but beautiful stretch of the Long Island coast. The purpose for this willed isolation was to produce poetry, art. Nearby lived a painter whose reputation was as esteemed as Pablo Picasso's. This unnamed male artist was rich, famous, gifted, and worked seven days a week: "What else is there to do?" he explained (13–14).

To Jordan, this brilliant man represented A Successful American and A Great Man. He was the kind of devoted artist she wanted to be. Day after day, she felt lucky to be where she was: writing poetry, walking along the seashore, and rarely answering her phone, as not many people called. It was not until she was raped, and had no one locally to call, that she realized the depravity of her isolation (13).[12]

The rape brought about a revelation: the model of the creative genius, the rugged individualist, not only is based on the privilege of white men but is a distorted model producing isolation and loneliness. "American delusions of individuality now disfigure our national landscape with multitudes of disconnected pained human beings who pull down the shades on prolonged and needless agony" (18). Jordan's longing for comfort and care in the wake of the rape alerted her to the disconnected life she was living.

Later, back in her own home in the suburbs, "living in an American-dream white cottage with tulips and hyacinth . . . inside that ideal, spotless, American house there is no one besides me and my answering machine and my VCR," Jordan once again recognized the remoteness of her life and the lives of those around her (21). Her landlord's wife rarely said hello. The wife's sole interaction with the world involved driving the family's jeep to the end of the driveway to retrieve the day's mail and then driving the jeep back to the house. Posted on the landlord's gate was a sign that read PRIVATE. Jordan believes that too many Americans, like the famous male artist of Long Island, are deluded into thinking that success means isolation and privacy means democracy. Jordan argues that democracy is not excessive individualism but a collective of people.

Jordan mourns the social costs of the cult of isolation. So much time is given to the idea that we must be "special" and "individuals" that we cannot empathize with other people's pain. If we only spoke openly about the injustices of our experiences we would begin to see our sameness and connection to others, and only then would we have a true democracy.

Like Jordan, Sherman also tells a story of how a black woman artist is deformed by a patriarchal conception of art, the artist, and society. Rayna's delusional state of mind is pierced by the trauma of testing positive. Assuming the role of the isolated artist tricks Rayna into a false sense of well-being, a well-being that is shattered when she tests positive. Rayna even wonders if she has used her art as an escape from the inevitable vulnerability of human intimacy and connection. But there is a crucial difference between Jordan and Sherman: Not once does Jordan conclude that because she succumbed to the propaganda of the isolated individual she should rethink her commitment to being an artist. Faced with the same insight as Rayna, Jordan uses her newfound knowledge as material for a poem and essay, while Rayna uses it against herself.[13]

Exposing the sterility and violence of the white male definition of the artist as one who ignores communal responsibility and human intimacy does not have to result in the recapitulation of selfless good woman. Jordan opens her essay with an excerpt from a poem about the very subject the essay will address: the American disease of delusional individuality. Rayna Sargent, however, increasingly shies away from her intense engagement with art, as if she is ashamed. Jordan relocates to the city and continues her work, while Rayna pits community service against the creation of art. Carving out the emotional and physical space to create art is not in and of itself a rejection of community service and human interaction, especially for black women who have been constructed as the mammies of the "serving" race.

Ironically, a male artist with AIDS in *touch*, Ricky Adonio, is presented as sensitive to community service; yet his burning desire to be an artist is never set against human connection. Ricky outlines how, with each new stage of physical deterioration, he invents a way to create:

> I kept painting until I couldn't do it anymore, then I started making bird-cages and selling them to nursing homes. Now I'm not strong enough to build the cages anymore, but I taught someone else to make them. The old people love the birds. . . . I saw myself moving through the four stages of

life. I wove what I saw into four wall hangings that I put up in my room. I get great peace from them.

Now I'm sick all the time. I try to go out and talk to the kids. Try to tell people about this disease. The talking gives me strength. (101–2)

While Rayna opens up to emotional support by eschewing what she calls "the crown worn by the cult of Strong Black Women" and becomes involved in a relationship and in community service, it is unfortunate that she increasingly sees her work as an artist as selfish and meaningless: "I've always been too into myself to care about spending a lot of time with somebody else. . . . I just can't see myself dying in a few years and all I'll have left behind is a roomful of painted canvases" (147, 182, 183). As tragic as it is that Rayna has tested positive, and as powerful as it is that she opens up to intimacy, support, and community service, it is equally tragic that she moves away from her lifelong passion to paint. In one of her early journal entries, Rayna writes, "When I burst out of my mother's womb, I was an artist. I know with all of my being that that is what I am and all that I ever want to be" (45).

touch presents a remarkably naive view of an inordinately complicated topic: communal mothering, sacrifice, gender roles, and female artistic identity in the age of epidemic. Sherman's novel opens with Rayna preparing for her first solo art show. Her friends complain that she spends much more time developing herself as an artist than in developing her relationships. While Rayna has two reliable, close female friendships, she has no lover, although she is not opposed to casual sex or to a long-term relationship. Rayna's women friends spend a great deal of time throughout the story questioning her serious engagement with her work. C'Anne barks, "Art isn't life," and focuses on Rayna's need for a relationship: "You gotta leave that art alone sometime and get out in the world" (28). She urges Rayna to call Theodore, the man with whom C'Anne thinks Rayna should become romantically involved. Both C'Anne and Novel feel that Rayna is too intense, and they do not understand her ongoing periods of paralysis followed by outbursts of productivity.

Later in the narrative, Theodore, who does become Rayna's boyfriend, also accuses Rayna of using her creativity as a "crutch." Although Sherman is aware of the centrality of Rayna's art to her autonomy and personal well-being, even after she tests positive, the author is at the same time cu-

riously unaware of how the voices of these subordinate characters trivial-
ize the main character's radical commitment to creative expression. It is as
if the text, like C'Anne, Novel, and Theodore, does not take Rayna's aspirations seriously.

Perhaps because of this, Rayna's artist's identity shrinks rather than ex-
pands in subsequent chapters. Rayna questions her identity as an artist
and takes on the mantle of communal mother, even though Sherman tells
us that art is "the most intimate part of [Rayna's] life" and has Rayna pro-
nounce, "art is my life" (28).

Rayna's movement away from an artist's life of solitude to a more communal life takes place gradually. First, her friend and fellow artist, Ricky,
is diagnosed with AIDS. Now that he is ill, Rayna feels guilty that she has
been socially withdrawn and preoccupied with painting and writes him a
brief letter. In the letter, she tells Ricky she loves him and that she doesn't
want him to be sick or to die. When Ricky contacts Rayna five months
later, she visits him at Bailey-Boushay House.

Then Rayna learns of the Briggs case. A psychiatrist at the hospital
where Rayna works tries to convince an HIV-positive black woman
named Latosha Briggs to have an abortion, but Latosha refuses. In response, one of the hospital's doctors sterilizes her without her consent.
The Prejudice Posse, a woman's political action group that advocates on
behalf of Briggs and all HIV-positive women, decides to stage a political
action at the hospital. Unwittingly, Rayna becomes one of the targets of
the action, which consists of a small group of women throwing a vial of
red liquid at her and a receptionist with the taunt, "We thought we'd
help you with your fear of AIDS-tainted blood" (37). Rayna does not
condone what happened to Latosha Briggs, but she doesn't approve of
the Posse's approach: "Is this the only way you can find to make your
point?" (41).

The Prejudice Posse approaches Rayna again, at a time when she is very
depressed because an art collector insulted her the night before at an art
show that included her work; he would consider buying one of her paintings only if he could cut it in half "in order to make it work with my collection in the blue room" (51). Feeling defeated, Rayna responds to one
member of the Prejudice Posse: "Rayna looked into the older woman's
eyes. She felt as if she were looking into her mother's eyes, into Circe's
eyes. There was a kindness there, a beauty and grace. She reached for the

woman's hand" (57). Rayna promises that she will think about how she can help the women's group vindicate Latosha Briggs, a promise Rayna will eventually fulfill with the help of Novel.

Up to this point in the narrative, Rayna has tried to escape the world so that she can concentrate on her art. Like the traditional male artist, Rayna has always put her art first; but Latosha Briggs, Ricky Adonio, and the Prejudice Posse are on her mind. Also, at the urgings of her friends, she has started a relationship with a man. Then Rayna tests positive, and all she can think about is illness and death from AIDS; she feels that her apartment is a "grave." Rayna retreats from all social contact and sinks into a deep depression. Eventually, she seeks out a counselor, who helps her disclose her status to her friends, family, and boyfriend. She even begins to attend a women's support group, made up of diverse women.

But what is striking is that once Rayna regains some stability in her life after the shock of testing HIV positive, she is pulled in the direction of caring for the needs of others at the expense of her art. Unlike Ricky, who says the worst part of having the virus is that it takes away his ability to paint, by the end of the novel Rayna acts as if there is something morally suspect about being a female artist.

After Rayna gathers up the courage to tell her boyfriend, Theodore, that she is HIV positive, one of his immediate responses is that she "do something." His advice is that Rayna volunteer to teach art to HIV-positive children and children living with AIDS. Theodore says, "Maybe that's the beauty of this disease. It will push us so far outside of ourselves that we'll finally see how connected we are with everybody else living in the world" (171).[14] With some trepidation, Rayna eventually finds herself at the Dancing Unicorn House, where Theodore, with Rayna's approval, has arranged for her to teach art to the children. Rayna uses the experience for her personal development as well as to perform community service, but she is clearly being put into the role of caretaker, an activity that takes her away from creating art. With the introduction of the character Anika, a child with AIDS, Rayna's sense of herself as an artist is almost completely lost.

Anika is an adorable ten-year-old girl who contracted HIV as a result of child sexual abuse. Living with a mother who traded sex for drugs, Anika was exposed to HIV when several infected men sexually abused her. Now Anika lives in an AIDS residence for children. As a newly diagnosed HIV-positive person herself, and as an adopted child who was taken away from an "incompetent" mother, Rayna is ambivalent about working with the children, especially the "motherless," sexually abused Anika, who is in the late stages of AIDS. After some avoidance, Rayna begins regular visits, teaches art to the kids, and befriends Anika, who, just before she dies, asks Rayna to be her "mother." Though Rayna "decided long ago she would never have enough of herself to give to anything other than her art," she agrees to be Anika's surrogate mother (195).

Rayna's involvement with the children at Unicorn House, and particularly with Anika, becomes increasingly time-consuming and intense, and subsequently she begins to question her lifelong preoccupation with making art. Near the end of the novel, Rayna admits to Novel and C'Anne that taking care of these children is more important than being an artist. Rayna says she doesn't "have much time for art anymore. . . . My life is filled with work and children. And Theodore" (201).

Luckily for Rayna, her friends do an about-face and strongly disagree with her plan to give up art. C'Anne responds with open disapproval: "You can use your art for healing if you want, healing yourself and others. Cutting yourself off from one of the things that has sustained you most in life seems ridiculous, and, frankly, overdramatic" (184). C'Anne and Novel remind her that making art is the core of who she is, and while caretaking and working with these children is vital and important work, so is her art. In this way, community service on behalf of children is set against Rayna's identity as an artist. The last scene of the novel depicts Rayna grieving at Anika's grave, with Novel and C'Anne showing up to give their friend support. Novel mentions the body art collaboration piece Rayna agreed to work on with her, but Rayna says, "I can't think about that now" (213).

Anika's request that Rayna be her surrogate mother and Rayna's willingness to go along with it suggest Sherman's awareness of how many black women give back to their communities through the care of black children. As Patricia Hill Collins puts it, black women "feel accountable to all the Black community's children" ("Black Women," 205). Such changes in Rayna's character suggest a strategic repudiation of the patriarchal, capitalistic, white cult of the isolated artist. Rayna achieves intimacy, community, and activism when she takes the job at Dancing Unicorn and agrees to mother Anika, even if for only a short time. In so doing, Rayna is also healing herself.[15]

But the changes that occur in Rayna's character also demonstrate how the HIV/AIDS epidemic emboldens and glorifies the nurturing woman. The pandemic has increased the amount of caring labor women are expected to perform—caring for sick family and community members, even when women are HIV infected or ill—and it creates a representational rationalization in which woman as caregiver is constructed as the inevitable and natural "answer" to the crisis of AIDS. Self-definition and self-determination, qualities routinely associated with men in literature and culture, are thwarted when women are socialized into martyred care.

Ironically, while Sherman incorporates several key experiences of black women and AIDS into her text, from sterilization abuse to safer sex, she seems not to consider how the figure of the child with AIDS undermines Rayna's individuality. As discussed in Chapter 3, women (and most infected children) are literally and symbolically hidden behind the cultural spectacle of the idealized dying (white) child. In contrast to the many AIDS narratives in circulation, the child with AIDS in this text does not overwhelm or dominate the text. Equally important, Sherman does not include the child's deathbed scene. Yet Sherman accepts the underlying structure of gendered caretaking and the ways in which the ill child is used to maintain it; in fact, her narrative glorifies it.

While it is possible to interpret the image of care in the novel in terms of political practices of mothering in black communities, the gendering of care in the HIV/AIDS crisis has detrimental effects on women of all races. The gendered mandate that women should caretake is one of the most fundamental ways in which women (and men) are slotted into rigid gender roles. Giving Rayna's character aspirations and dreams, especially as an HIV-positive black artist, is an imaginative defense against the prevailing trivialization of women's struggle for self-definition and equality. When the narrative undermines Rayna's artist's identity, *touch* enacts, rather than challenges, the themes of women and care found in medical, political, and cultural discourses on AIDS.

As a result, a female character with HIV infection is subordinated, once again, to a supposedly "larger," less selfish perspective, and Sherman loses "touch" with the significance of Rayna's power as a woman who exists for herself and not only for the caretaking of others. An underlying message of *touch* is that when HIV/AIDS enters a woman's life, regardless of her own health status, certain "feminine" behaviors are expected. The anxiety, fears, and stigmas revived by a sexual health epidemic such as HIV drive many women to adopt conservative, conventional ideas of female agency, and Sherman's Rayna is no exception. Instead of suggesting that HIV/AIDS offers Rayna a new basis for self-development *and* community, *touch* underscores that "a woman who insists on equity seems heartless" (Valian, 43).

Push

Echoing Alice Walker's epistolary format in *The Color Purple*, Sapphire's *Push*, like *touch*, uses the main female character's journal entries to address the themes of mother-daughter as well as father-daughter incest, and the topics of poverty, sexuality, welfare reform, and education from the perspectives of diverse girl characters, including a young butch lesbian. But the bulk of the short novel concerns the main character, a young black girl named Precious Jones, who becomes a poet, a mother, and HIV positive by the time she is sixteen years old. For many readers, critics, and reviewers, such a plot and focus are too much; for Sapphire, the novel transforms some of the author's experiences of teaching young black girls in Harlem into art.

Unlike *touch*, *Push* has been the subject of enormous controversy. According to Michelle Cliff, *Push* signals Sapphire's sellout to white capitalism because she received a $250,000 advance against royalties. Dale Peck, a white gay man, asserts that the novel "is terrible" and "virtually unreadable"(quoted in Hamburger, 23). To one young reviewer in New York City's *New Youth Connections*, the book reinforces racial and gender stereotypes by making the main character seem "like an incompetent fool" and an "imbecile" (Grey, 19). Ethelbert Miller offers an alternative reading: "If you get past [the strong language of *Push*], you'll see that [Sapphire is] addressing some very important issues" (quoted in Bailey).

Reminiscent of the critical reaction to Alice Walker's *The Color Purple*, *Push* has been rejected by some as "a tool of white people" intent on showing "a dysfunctional view of the black family" (Bell-Scott, 80). Hortense Spillers was so moved by the controversy surrounding the novel that she organized a panel on the topic of contemporary black women's fiction for the 1997 Modern Language Association meeting. One paper on the Spillers panel carried a revealing title: "Authenticity as Commodity in Contemporary Black Women's Literature." The hype and publicity surrounding *Push* led Spillers to question why representations of black women's and girls' pain are so profitable.

Push is an underdeveloped yet extremely important novel, because it approaches HIV infection in black girls in terms of incest. In a sense, Sapphire's text emerges as a literary tracking of the link between sexual assault and HIV infection in girls and serves as a direct challenge to the Centers for Disease Control's continued trivialization of sexual assault and HIV infection in children.[16] *Push* may indeed be misused or appropriated by white racists; and the controversy surrounding its publication clearly indicates the need for extensive, critical discussion of why representations of African American girls' and women's pain function in a voyeuristic manner in our culture. But such critical conversations, while long overdue, need not drown out or overshadow Sapphire's achievement in breaking silence on an issue no one wants to address. As bell hooks reminds us, "critical interrogation is not the same as dismissal," and so raising critical questions about the novel does not rule out what is powerful about it (*Teaching,* 49).

In graphic detail, Sapphire delineates, among other things, the sexual and emotional violence that Precious Jones endures at the hands of her disturbed, sadistic parents, whose behavior toward their daughter is never explained. Precious's parents may have had a tough childhood, but that is no excuse for the way they treat their daughter. *Push* has little patience for the worlds of social work, public health care, and public education, populated as they are in this fiction with indifferent, unethical characters who are black and white, male and female. Instead, *Push* directs its angry gaze at the family and community of Precious Jones. Not interested in promulgating a positive black family or community image as the key to emancipation, and not concerned with how white readers will use the narrative it tells against black people, *Push* exposes father-mother-daughter incest, homophobia, and the seriousness of HIV in the context of gender and race as systemic institutions. Precious eventually has to wrestle with a disease that she thinks is naturally associated with "white faggits" and "crack addicts," and part of her struggle includes facing her own learned homophobia and internalized racism and sexism.[17]

Midway through the novel, Precious begins to write poetry at the same time that she learns that she has contracted HIV from forced sex with her father. Precious's reaction to this news, as recorded in her journal, is a skillful debunking of the racial assumptions of white women's suffering as depicted in mainstream AIDS discourse: "I don't want to cry. I tell myself I WILL NOT cry when I am writing, 'cause number one I stop writing and number two I just don't always want to be crying like white bitch on TV movies" (127). In the context of women and AIDS, sentimentality may be used to break silences, and it may even be used to make legible the experiences of HIV-positive women; but Sapphire's Precious, similar to Barbara Neely's Blanche White, exposes sentimentality's self-serving privileging of white women's tears. Providing her girl character with inner strength and artistic desires, Sapphire honors perseverance, self-definition, and creative exploration as central themes in black women's literary texts, and, significantly, she locates these in young women characters living with HIV.[18]

The disappointment in *Push*, as in *touch*, stems from its overall retreat from an in-depth development of the main characters. Ironically, the main characters in both texts never move beyond shadowy individualities, despite the use of the personal journal device. By not allowing Precious a radical individuality, the novel unwittingly duplicates the patronizing and emblematic use of women in dominant representations of AIDS. Although *touch* does this more often than *Push* does, both novels sometimes recapitulate the predominant conception of women and girls as secondary beings who are inevitably defined by someone else or through the structure of sentimental nurture and racial imagery.

As Lisa Kennedy points out, *Push* is more interested in exploring the well-established themes of monstrosity and invisibility, themes found in such classic male texts as Richard Wright's *Native Son* and Ralph Ellison's *Invisible Man*, than in offering a detailed development of her characters' interior lives (76). *Push*'s "abbreviated" characterizations of Precious, the other young black women in Precious's literacy class, and her mentor, Ms. Rain, remain within the prevailing gender and race representations of women in general and in AIDS discourse in particular (Gomez, 82). Furthermore, Precious's journal entries record her determination and initiative, but often the voice and language attributed to her shift so inexplicably that Precious doesn't sound like herself. In addition, the other crucial characters who supposedly foster Precious's self-definition—as she fosters theirs—are out of focus (Gomez).

In order to understand how Precious changes from an illiterate, overweight incest survivor into a budding poet and caring mother of two children—one with Down's Syndrome—spawned by her brutal father, it would also help to understand how her teacher, Ms. Rain, an out black lesbian, reaches her when all of the adults in Precious's life, particularly her warped parents and teachers, have failed her miserably. Yet we never see the process of Precious's emerging literacy, and it is as if she miraculously overcomes the embedded systems of race and gender through individual willpower and commitment. The ferocity of Precious's hunger for self-expression and her difficult struggle to engage in the demanding process of intellectual-creative labor demand much more space than they are given.

Sapphire's novel does come closer than Sherman's to externalizing the politics of the theme of self-definition, largely because *Push* stays closely focused on Precious's journal entries and includes the writings of Precious's classmates at the novel's end. But the reader is deprived of the inner lives of these characters as they maintain and/or resist the institutions of gender and race. Sapphire's purpose seems to be to develop the impact of a woman-hating, racist, homophobic culture on her girl character, and, at the same time, to create a character who cannot be reduced to the contrived talk-show labels: "incest survivor," "HIV-positive teenager," "unwed, young, black teenage mother on welfare." Sapphire wants to make Precious more than a collection of "social ills." But she fails to do so, and thus fails Precious and the other characters in the book.

Giving her characters the space and time they need to create their own self-defined individualities might have helped Sapphire in her effort to expose the brutal effects of multiple oppressions. This lack of development shifts the narrative toward the genre of slick, superficial, tabloid story—a genre that tends to work with dominant race and gender ideologies rather than against them. Since Sapphire correctly suggests that AIDS and incest are not "private" issues, what is needed in *Push* is a longer, more developed novel, so that the characters' development matches the "bigness" of the novel's social themes (Gomez, 82).

Most problematically, the novel demonstrates Precious's hard-won struggle to create an independent poet's identity, while at the same time romanticizing her biological motherhood. As poet and critic Cheryl Clarke argues, motherhood operates as a "smokescreen" in this novel behind which smolders Precious's tender desire for autonomy and artistic self-definition (38). Clarke writes, "I much prefer Precious's newly acquired poet's identity" to her "overdetermined maternal identity," but Precious's poet's identity is subordinate to her identity as devoted mother (38). Perhaps an unwed, young black mother deserves maternal idealization rather than the relentless denigration heaped on her in America. Nevertheless, Ms. Rain raises some important questions about the privileging of motherhood that are never answered. In a written back-and-forth dialogue with Precious, Ms. Rain challenges Precious's contention that without Precious's "angel child" she "don't have nothing" (72, 142). In response to this claim, Ms. Rain writes, "It seems the opposite to me. If you keep Abdul you might have nothing. You are learning to read and write, that is everything" (142). The point is that the tension and contradiction around motherhood and autonomy for a young black woman are never fully fleshed out. It is as if the tainted Precious were being redeemed through her role as self-sacrificing mother, a familiar ploy operating in much AIDS discourse on women.

Happy Endings

As in *touch* and *Push*, the controversial topics of AIDS and sexuality in African American communities are remarkably realized in Pearl Cleage's *What Looks Like Crazy on an Ordinary Day.* Included in Oprah's Book Club and loved by readers across the country, the novel uses a straightforward, sarcastic, and humorous style to recount the story of Ava Johnson, an independent, clear-thinking African American woman who tests HIV positive and decides to "do the right thing": write letters to her former sexual partners suggesting that they get tested, too. Once the missives are sent, Ava is bombarded with negative response from members of her chic, high-powered community in Atlanta. She receives a visit from an enraged wife who wants to know "what you think you're doing sending my husband some shit like this through the mail" (8). Snubbed by all and forced to sell her lucrative hair salon and attractive home, Ava makes plans to relocate to San Francisco, the most HIV-positive-friendly city in the world. However, before moving to San Francisco, Ava returns to her hometown of Idlewild, Michigan, to spend the summer with her widowed sister, Joyce Mitchell, with whom she enjoys a close and open relationship.

With diary entries as chapters, the narrative begins with Ava's reasons for journeying to Idlewild and what she finds when she gets there. Once an African American lake resort in northern Michigan that flourished in the 1950s and 1960s, Idlewild is now in economic and social decline. Ava's entries refer to such problems as gangs, drugs, teenage pregnancy, domestic violence, sexism, poor education, and high unemployment—big-city problems in a small lakeside town. These various subjects are intertwined with entries about Ava's feelings about testing HIV positive, her unexpected attraction to a character named Eddie Jefferson, and the conservative (and deadly) maneuvers of the New Light Baptist Church.

The action begins when Eddie, a friend of Joyce's and Joyce's deceased husband, meets Ava at the airport because Joyce is rushing a pregnant teenager to the hospital where the young woman, who is HIV positive and crack-addicted, gives birth. (This birth will have a profound effect on all the characters' lives.) The attraction between Ava and Eddie is believably and sensually rendered over the course of the novel, with the two characters confessing their love midway. The sexual romance convincingly occurs within the context of the three main characters' experiences in the community as they confront, separately and collectively, the multiple problems in the town.

Despite the grave issues the characters encounter, *What Looks Like Crazy* willfully and strategically ends happily with the marriage of Ava and Eddie; the return of Imani (the baby born to the HIV-positive, crack-addicted teen) to Joyce; the installment of a new, enlightened female pastor, replacing the conservative Reverend Anderson, who turns out to be an alcoholic and pederast; the success of the Sewing Circus, a support group for young African American women managed mostly by Joyce; and the enrollment of Aretha, an orphaned teenager, in an expensive, private, arts-centered high school. Cleage's use of romance and a happy ending defies the typical image of HIV-positive women as defective, abject, dirty victims who must forgo romantic love. Such an ending also offers an alternative vision of racial uplift, one rooted in openness about sex rather than stifling respectability.[19]

A critique of ladylike silence as defense is fleshed out in the scene in which Ava's sister, Joyce, is demonstrating safer sex techniques to the young women's support group by applying a condom to a hot dog, and then is verbally attacked by Mrs. Gerry Anderson, the reverend's wife, for teaching young women how to sexually stimulate men. These young teenage mothers engage in unsafe, unsatisfying, and often unwanted sex with domineering and abusive boyfriends, and Joyce is determined to empower them. Yet Mrs. Anderson interprets the group's workshop on sexual health as corrupt and indecent. Such a response reveals Mrs. Anderson as a sexually repressed, ultraconservative church lady trapped in outdated ideology: "She was wearing a pale blue polyester pantsuit and white sandals with stockings. Her hair, which was pressed and hot-curled within an inch of its life, was elaborately styled and piled like Mahalia Jackson's when she sang her solo at the end of *Imitation of Life*. Hardly anybody asks for that kind of hard press anymore. Sister seems to have missed the moment when we decided it was okay for the hair to *move*" (50–51).

Anderson's demeanor and self-righteousness are doubly ironic since her husband, the Reverend Anderson, surfaces in Idlewild because of sexual abuse allegations in his former clergy post in Chicago. Cleage concocts such a plot to hammer home the hypocrisy of moral self-righteousness. When Joyce declares that Mrs. Anderson is "out of touch," Cleage is questioning Anderson's version of ladylike racial uplift in the age of twin epidemics: AIDS and drugs (79). The novel proposes that those who vociferously protest any discussion of sex outside heterosexual Christian marriage are suffering from sexual repression or trying to conceal, in the case of Mrs. Anderson's husband, sexual violence.

Like *touch* and *Push*, *What Looks Like Crazy* dismantles many of the stereotypical assumptions associated with AIDS, such as that the illness afflicts only certain groups and that all HIV-positive people—with some exceptions—are guilty: "If you're not a little kid, or a heterosexual movie star's doomed but devoted wife, or a hemophiliac who got it from a tainted transfusion, or a straight white woman who can prove she's a virgin with a dirty dentist, you're not eligible for any no-strings sympathy" (4). Here Cleage is referring directly to some of the acceptable, high-profile media figures with AIDS: Ryan White, Elizabeth Glaser, and Kimberly Bergalis.

Cleage's novel repeatedly argues that misconceptions and bigoted narratives about women and AIDS stem from deep conflicts over sexuality.

For instance, Ava Johnson's assessment of a group of women with AIDS on a TV talk show deconstructs the good girl/bad girl dichotomy to which many HIV-positive women cling: "There they were, weeping and wailing and wringing their hands, wearing their prissy little Laura Ashley dresses and telling their edited-for-TV life stories. . . . They get diagnosed and all of a sudden they're Mother Teresa" (3). By providing her main character with a quick wit, romance, and sex, Cleage offers a powerful challenge to the Mother Teresa syndrome.

But like the other two novels, Cleage's book participates in a seeming (and naive) validation of the mythic narrative of woman as natural care-giver. *What Looks Like Crazy* depicts an HIV-negative character, Ava's sister, Joyce Mitchell, as the one who uncomplainingly performs an endless amount of good works and services: "Anybody with trouble knew if they could get to Joyce she'd take care of it" (14). Joyce's character is the devotional mother icon incarnate. Years after Joyce's two children have died, and two years after her husband has been killed in a tragic accident, Joyce is understandably still depressed, overweight, and lost. In this mind-set, she receives a phone call that Ava is HIV positive. Joyce rushes to Atlanta and encourages Ava to come back home for the summer. Over the course of the novel, Joyce attends to the needs of her sister, Ava; the troubled young women who attend Joyce's support group (they begin holding meetings at Joyce's house when the group loses its space at the church); the old people in town whose homes are being burglarized; and the crack baby who is abandoned by one of the teenagers (after its birth, the baby comes to live with Joyce and is later taken away and then returned with its legs broken). Joyce also must respond to vicious attacks and opposition from Mrs. Gerry Anderson over the activities of the Sewing Circus, help Aretha, the orphaned teenager, apply to a competitive summer program, and file a complaint against teenagers who throw a rock through her front window (the teens turn out to be Mrs. Gerry Anderson's grandson and a friend). Often, Ava or Eddie assists in these activities, but the language of the novel makes it clear that Joyce is the one who does most of the work.

Throughout the novel, Joyce is presented as a brave activist. Fighting injustice gives her life meaning—especially in light of her many losses.[20] A former state caseworker, Joyce is now after fifteen years free from the bureaucratic quagmire of the social work industry and able to really help people better their lives. She does accomplish this, miraculously without any detriment to her physical and emotional health, thus winning the admiration of her sister, Eddie, and the reader. But surely the dangerous stress that comes with a workload such as Joyce's takes its toll on her body and mind, and this is one of the novel's subtle silences.

However, figuring an HIV-negative woman, rather than an HIV-positive woman, as the uncomplaining caretaker breaks a common pattern in representations of women and AIDS. In addition, Joyce's character exists alongside a less traditional conception of sacrifice and care, as Ava expresses gentle sarcasm about Joyce's tendency to "fix" everything.

Ava offers an alternative model as she fashions her own mode of care. Before joining in the service work with which Joyce is engaged, Ava takes time to adjust to being back home. Cleage has her character taking long naps in the sun, like a sleepy, calm cat; learning how to meditate; and enjoying long morning walks by the lake and picnics with Eddie. Again, Ava refuses to be Mother Teresa like the HIV-positive women she sees on talk shows try to do (3). But she also thinks about the problems besetting her sister and her hometown, and decides that helping to take care of the crack baby, helping to administer the Sewing Circus, and fighting conservative, AIDS-phobic Christians are meaningful, self-actualizing activities. These activities allow her to experience self-love and community at a time when she feels she has neither, and to witness young African American women emerging in strength and power.

Because Ava's caretaking is never done in isolation and because she experiences romance and sex, her character seems empowered rather than depleted by the volunteer work. Through Ava, Cleage resists the self-sacrificing devotional mother icon as a surefire way to redeem an HIV-positive woman.

Through Ava, Cleage also explores oppression and domination within marginalized communities. Ava's perspective on the black community, on AIDS, and on sexuality—including queer sexuality—is not commonly found within the dominant culture or within black communities. With a shrewd eye for hypocrisy and contradiction, Ava points out the harmfulness of puritanical attitudes toward sex, homophobic ideology, and rigid family structure to the black community's health and survival. The narrative even looks at the negative impact of rigid gender roles on young black men. Tyrone, one of the young black male teenagers, who rapes and beats his girlfriend and then encourages his friend to rape her too, is the grandson of the Andersons. Part of what has contributed to Tyrone's dysfunction is the fact that his own mother died of AIDS and his Christian grandparents refuse to talk about it.

Cleage contrasts Tyrone's masculinity with an alternative black masculinity embodied in the character of Eddie, a man who was once like the violent young men who terrorize the lake community. A reformed man, Eddie practices a gentle, peaceful, respectful life after years of "death energy": Vietnam, the drug world, and being in prison for committing murder. When Ava meets Eddie, he is a Buddhist who practices tai chi, drinks tea, and is a vegetarian. The relationship Eddie creates with Ava is erotic, emotionally open, loving, and promising. Eddie's past and present life suggest the character's shift from traditional hypermasculinity to a "softer" masculinity. Eddie symbolizes a new masculinity, a replacement for the rigid roles of subordinate woman and patriarchal man.[21]

Selfless, caretaking black woman is a potent expression of mythic womanhood. In *touch*, caretaking entails a subtle belittlement of Rayna Sargent's artistic identity. In *Push* it entails an overdetermined physical, as opposed to metaphoric, motherhood. In *What Looks Like Crazy* gendered care is displaced onto the HIV-negative older sister. All three novels use interior devices such as journal and diary entries, and all three grapple with dominant ideas of women as didactic symbols of moral sacrifice and care.[22] Thus, in addition to initiating a black feminist literary intervention into the realm of HIV, these narratives tell us something about representation and gender in the age of AIDS. They produce contradictions that draw attention to the tenacity of gendered ideology at the heart of representations of AIDS and thus to the constructedness of "woman."

What these novels suggest is that women in the United States have struggled with historical and cultural narratives of race, gender, and sexuality for centuries. While differences among women have made this struggle more difficult for some than for others, all women have had to struggle for the right to develop and practice multifaceted individualities and sexual self-determination. An analysis of the linkages between women and AIDS in representation suggests that, given the entrenched institution of gender, this basic human right has yet to be fully accomplished anywhere.[23]

The conflation of women with sacrifice in these novels does not undermine their important literary and political contributions. Each narrative uses women's journals and letters to integrate the conflicted, painful experiences of women and girls into AIDS discourse, and initiating the theme of AIDS into black feminist literary traditions could save women's lives. Progressive texts that speak out on women and HIV, even if these same texts subtly reproduce gendered ideologies, are still preferable to silence.

CONCLUSION

BEYOND SENTIMENTAL AIDS

All the textual and visual representations of women and AIDS that I have been analyzing recall Hilton Als's discussion of the black woman as "Negress," an identity he links to American culture's historical roots in what he calls "puritanical selflessness" (7). Puritanical selflessness links "the Negress" with the "good woman" construct so prevalent in AIDS.[1] Just as the Negress is a "good," strong, black woman—"selfless to a fault"—so is she (along with the generic white "good woman") a prevailing conception that structures many representations of women and AIDS (Als, 8). By and large, women's puritanical self-abnegation is the bedrock of narratives and visual culture on AIDS.

But fortunately, some discourse on women and AIDS refuses to reproduce the mammy/good woman paradigm. In addition to Cleage's *What Looks Like Crazy on an Ordinary Day*, Tiye Milan Selah's short story "An Elegy for Jade" addresses many of the real problems black women with HIV and AIDS encounter—invisibility, ignorance, and lack of care linked to historically entrenched racism and sexism. It also forcefully abandons the idealized sacrificial woman as solution and device.

"An Elegy for Jade" presents a woman character with AIDS, Jade, through the admiring eyes of her best friend, Leilani. Both characters are self-possessed, creative black women linked together through a long friendship. Through Leilani's point of view, we learn about Jade's experiences as an HIV-positive woman.

When the story opens, Jade has sent Leilani an envelope filled with letters addressed to Jade's former lovers; each note is identical and includes a Yoruba poem as well as an anonymous message written by Jade, encouraging the recipient of the letter to get tested. There is also a note for Leilani: "Leilani, I really feel that this is the best way to handle warning my past lovers. Anonymously. I thank you in advance for your help. Eternally, Jade" (114). Leilani mails the envelopes on her way out for her morning run.

From the start, this story differs from the prevailing representation of black women and AIDS: both women are presented as fully developed individuals, actively expressing themselves through creative expression, business plans, and intellect. Though Leilani lives in Philadelphia and Jade in Minneapolis/St. Paul, they have helped each other cope with corporate glass ceilings just as they have cultivated each other's ambitions, dreams, plans, and desires. Jade's undergraduate and advanced degrees in chemistry and international marketing have meant extensive travel, allowing her to discover that her true dream "was to cultivate a perfume line, using the exotic scents of indigenous flowers from regions all over the world" (115). And Leilani, a "master gemologist," discloses to Jade that she would like to open her own "jewelry store featuring exclusive ethnically crafted fine jewelry" (115). As Leilani explains, she and Jade are true artists, always "preparing for a new type of self-expression" (115). Similar to Sherman's Rayna Sargent, Selah's characters are artistic black women.

We also see a clear delineation of care as a central issue in AIDS. Jade is experiencing an "exile" from family and friends and undergoing long periods of loneliness and isolation. Although she attends a support group and receives other services from an AIDS organization in her city, the programs rendered are created with white gay men in mind: "Services addressing the needs of American women of African descent were not offered in her area" (114). Jade attends an African American community-based organization and encounters different, yet equally serious, problems: the services available are pitched to IV drug users, mothers, and children. Jade discovers that "[s]he did not fit into [the] categories"; she does not match the prescribed narratives of women and AIDS (120).

It was to Leilani, rather than the women in her family, that Jade turned five years earlier when she first became ill. Jade explained to Leilani that her female relatives had "spent so much time consoling others, being brave, neglecting their own needs, being *strong black women*" that she felt she could not turn to them for care; Jade felt she would be a burden (114). When Leilani considers Jade's isolation and difficulty, she poses a question to herself and to the reader: "Where is the village?" The black women in Jade's family are worn out from being *strong black women;* the AIDS service organization doesn't address her friend's needs. Leilani and Jade's grandmother, Miss Ginger Rose, willingly drive from Philadelphia to the Twin Cities to care for Jade, but Jade has borne much of this illness alone. Leilani's question, "Where is the village?" actively exposes care as one of the most important issue of AIDS. While neither Leilani nor the story can answer the question of who cares, the story does make clear the seriousness of the question and vociferously argues against "good woman" as an answer.

Furthermore, "An Elegy for Jade" develops a historical perspective by showing how African Americans fared in past epidemics and how they are faring now in the age of AIDS epidemic. The author compares Jade's experiences with HIV infection to her ancestors' infections with tuberculosis, illustrating that illness and racism are institutional problems, not "personal problems" that can be dismissed as bad luck or a fact of nature.

In the course of their journey from Philadelphia to the Twin Cities, Leilani asks Miss Ginger Rose about Jade's mother, Eva, and this one question unravels connections between Jade's experience with infection and that of her ancestors. Miss Ginger Rose explains how she, Jade's mother, and her great-grandmother all contracted tuberculosis at the pottery factory where they were employed (and exploited). In those days, news of a family's infection resulted in a visit from the police, who would post a "QUARANTINE" sign on the home and then send the "sick" family to another city or town (118).

Ginger Rose also recounts the difficulties black people had finding treatment.[2] She tells tales of Philadelphia hospitals that kept beds empty rather than make them available to African Americans. She talks of Dr. Henry Minton from South Carolina who opened the "Henry Phipps Institute's Negro Clinic" in response to the health crisis. And finally, she remembers how Jade's mother, Eva, became a nurse because of the impact tuberculosis had on her family and community, and how as a nurse she contracted the disease on the job (118).

In listening to Ginger Rose's story, Leilani recalls Jade's telling her that she has suffered TB "associated with AIDS," a memory that further emphasizes the author's desire to bring the past and the present together (120). Unlike Harriet Beecher Stowe's Little Eva, whose illness is taken out of history—a telltale sign of sentimentalization, argues Gayle Pemberton (279)—Jade's illness is woven into a narrative of AIDS, TB, institutional racism, and family history.

In the last section of the story, Leilani and Ginger Rose finally arrive in Minneapolis, where they learn that Jade has been in the hospital for three weeks "and in intensive care in a coma for the past three days" (121). They administer care by massaging Jade, talking to her, and waiting. When Leilani goes to Jade's apartment to rest, she discovers "two prototypes of perfumes, one labeled Ginger Rose, and the other Leilani" (122). Jade also prepared advertising campaigns for the new perfumes. Next to this work, Jade left an envelope, "complete with power of attorney instructions for [Leilani] and directives for her physicians" (122). Leilani and Miss Ginger Rose will make decisions about Jade's care and death based on these documented wishes.

While "An Elegy for Jade" focuses primarily on women characters coming to terms with another woman's inevitable death from AIDS, it also functions as a communal elegy for all black women whose bodies and lives have been, and will be, affected. It uses the so-called breakdown attributed to HIV / AIDS as an opportunity for social critique, historical connection, and artistic expression rather than for the solidification of dominant cultural narratives. It eschews the "good woman" not only by confronting epidemics but by exposing the broad, institutional narratives that lie ready to emerge in times of social unrest.

All the written and visual materials I have discussed share one aspect: they expose (if only inadvertently) the injustice of the sacrificial paradigm and lend themselves to a critical illumination of the power of controlling narratives. As Deborah Silverton Rosenfelt suggests, representational "structures reveal rather than forcibly resolve the contradictions in our lives" (147). These materials reveal that a powerful narrative about what counts as a valuable, good woman animates our current public and private discourse on AIDS.

NOTES

Preface

1. As Pia Thielmann points out, the danger of "the symbol 'Mother / Woman' " is that it "makes real flesh-and-blood women an abstraction, even if it's an elevating abstraction" (64).

2. Sarah Schulman similarly discusses the problematic visibility of lesbians in Jonathan Larson's *Rent*.

3. See Odets.

4. For work on women and AIDS from a global perspective, see Long and Ankrah; and Berer with Ray.

Chapter 1. Women and AIDS

1. See Golden.

2. See Valian, who uses the term "gender schema" to refer to historically entrenched ideas about gender embedded in people and institutions. Gender schemas are "cognitive frameworks" (104).

3. Carol Levine writes, "I was labeled a 'selfish wife,' since I refused to take [my husband] home without home care" (1588).

4. For a different view on heterosexual women, gay men, and AIDS in drama, see Fierstein. The main female character contracts HIV from her closeted ex-husband while her ex-husband's lover tests negative.

Another interesting departure is Jane Gillooly's documentary film on abortion, which is an unusual linking of women's health and sexuality to that of gay men. In *Leona's Sister, Gerri* (1995), Gillooly explores the true story of a young, white, working-class woman who died in a motel of an illegal abortion in 1964. Near the end of the film, Gillooly makes a visual connection to the sexuality and health of gay men in the AIDS epidemic when she focuses her lens on a white gay man dressed in a priest's robes as he marches in an AIDS Coalition to Unleash Power (ACT UP) demonstration. A large wooden cross rests on his left shoulder; in his right hand is a poster with an enlarged photo of the dead Geraldine Santoro—the subject of Gillooly's film—bloodied, nude, and hunched over. The ACT UP chant, "Act Up! Fight Back! Fight AIDS," appears in black letters underneath the Santoro image.

Gillooly's focus on the gay man carrying the gruesome photo of Santoro (which was taken by state medical examiners and somehow leaked to reporters and feminist writers) suggests a point of convergence of sexual politics, reproductive freedom, and the politics of health. The photo's appearance in an "AIDS" setting seems as inevitable as in a pro-choice rally in Washington, D.C., for Santoro's untimely death resulted from some of the same factors that have led to the deaths of so many people in the AIDS epidemic: the demonization of sexual activity outside of heterosexual marriage; social policies that punish, control, and restrict people's bodies and sexuality; and inadequate health care.

Factors involved in the literary-critical silence on women and AIDS are complex, but they clearly relate to the logic of traditional gender roles. Thomas Piontek writes that literary representations of the epidemic have received little critical attention from cultural critics (131). Contemporary novels, poetry, plays, and memoirs on HIV are not viewed as "academic literature" by most professors of English; Tony Kushner's play, a Pulitzer Prize winner, serves as one of the few exceptions. Piontek's explanation for this professional silence is homophobia, yet he is unusual in offering insight on the critical and literary silence on women and AIDS. He says this silence can be found in the history of women's oppression. As Piontek points out, "While women historically have been excluded from education and publishing, [white] homosexual men have had access to literary production by virtue of their gender privilege" (134).

Stuart Marshall shows the intersection between homophobia and sexism by discussing at length the medicalized identities of gay men and women. He points to the conjunction between the rise of photography and the construction of deviant social identities by the medical community. Deviancy was ascribed to persons who engaged in or exhibited a variety of "antisocial" behaviors: homosexuality, prostitution, alcoholism, hysteria, or madness. Here Marshall demonstrates the overlapping experiences between gay men and "deviant" women. The "medicalization" of women, and of homosexual men, was, and still is, a form of social control of "threatening" sexuality. Marshall limits his discussion to the tendency to use the crisis of AIDS to remedicalize the identity of the gay man. But the irony arises when Marshall challenges the construction of AIDS as a gay male disease (he points to the original acronym of AIDS as GRID, gay related immune disease, as an echo of early medical biological determinism), and yet fails to imagine how such a construction affects women. Women and feminism are evoked in order to recognize experiential connections, but then they are dropped in Marshall's AIDS representational theory.

The *New York Times Magazine* published two leading articles on "the end of AIDS" in the fall of 1996, both from a white gay male perspective. There is nothing wrong with publishing articles on AIDS from a white gay male perspective, yet it is worrisome that this standpoint alone continues to prevail in the *Times* and elsewhere. In one article, Andrew Sullivan explains that AIDS isn't just a gay male crisis, a point he often makes when confronted with right-wing homophobia; but then he explores AIDS solely in terms of its effects on masculinity, gay male sexuality, and cultural responses to male homosexuality—as if these categories exist in a closed circle and have absolutely no effect on other social realities. Women, African Americans, Latinas—as Sullivan suggests—are too abject and pathetic prior to testing HIV positive to be perceived as victims worthy of the language of tragedy. The *Magazine* has yet to publish an article on AIDS by an HIV-positive black gay man or a female sex worker or a black heterosexual woman visual artist or a lesbian immigrant or a white suburban woman who resists being constructed in terms of "immaculate infection."

5. Cindy Patton explains that the conflation of HIV/AIDS with social outcasts has led to the invention of "nominal queers." Even white middle-class housewives, children, and conservative grandmothers—identities not commonly possessing a preexisting outsider stigma—can slip into the category of "queer" by virtue of testing HIV positive: "Once perceptions of HIV risk were linked to social deviance, literally anyone, or any category of people deemed epidemiologically significant could be converted into nominal queers" (19). I am extending Patton's idea by arguing that the figure of traditional white femininity is used to mediate this "queering" process, not only in mass media, but in progressive artistic and popular discourses as well. HIV-positive "queer" woman redeems herself by acting on the good woman as caretaker mandate. Also, as Patton points out, despite the fact that HIV-positive women may become "queer," they are routinely constructed as secondary to the dominant position of "queer" men (111–12).

6. I am less interested in tabulating the numbers of absences or presences of women in various AIDS discourses than in how the social construction of "woman" is inadvertently "set up as a smokescreen to protect detested communities from the public gaze" (Gorna, 29). As Robin Gorna proposes, women are used as a moral shield. At the same time, women, as a class, are marginalized in patriarchal structures (37). A monitoring of AIDS discourse provides a fairly reliable reading of what inevitably counts as acceptable "woman" in patriarchal Western culture. Despite feminist gains, "woman" is still white, middle-class, heterosexual, and a mother.

7. See Wood; Golden. Although Wood's research does not focus on AIDS, her analysis of the social construction of care was instrumental in my interpretation of women in print and visual AIDS culture. Also, for a lesbian perspective on caregiving (a viewpoint absent from much of the literature on women and care), see DeLombard.

8. These statistics are based on information published in the Centers for Disease Control's July 1997 "CDC Update" and in an article by the National Congressional Black Caucus, published in *World* in June 1998. The reason women's experiences and perspectives have been absent from AIDS discourse is that such experiences and perspectives are still routinely excluded from historical events. As Patty Reagan writes, "It took longer for women's voices and realities to be included in the discourse on AIDS because events of historical significance have traditionally been given to men in power to judge, appropriate, and critique" (155).

9. Protease inhibitors can cost up to $20,000 a year, preventing many people who test positive (and do not have health insurance) from receiving treatment. Other drawbacks of protease inhibitors include an extremely strict drug schedule; serious, physically deforming side effects; and ineffective response, which can lead to resistant strains of HIV.

10. Proposing that a complex relationship between representation, language, and reality exists does not mean that material reality does not exist. As Julia T. Wood argues, concern with matters of representation and with the symbolic function of language "is sometimes misrepresented as an argument that there is no 'real reality.' Understanding the formative power of language, however, does not require assuming there is no empirical world. Instead, this perspective simply assumes that the meaning or significance of the experiences and ideas is neither absolute nor given. Because social values inhere in symbols, children, in acquiring language, simultaneously inherit the values and assumptions of the social order into which they are born" (124).

11. For further discussion of this idea, see Patton, 1–7.

12. In a May 1997 issue of the Rutgers University undergraduate student newspaper, the *Daily Targum*, an article appearing under the rubric of "AIDS awareness" constructs a young black woman with HIV infection as a vengeful temptress. The author tells the story of "a slender, no-nonsense Black woman . . . who attended several of my family's get-togethers: Christmas Eve dinners, Fourth of July barbecues and birthday parties" (14). A year later, the author learns that this "no-nonsense" young woman whom he had brought into his own home subsequently contracted HIV infection from her boyfriend, a college football player. Her response to the news was to seek revenge by "having sex with various members of the football team. She revealed her HIV status to her partners in the team's locker room at the end of the season; later, several of her partners developed HIV as well" (14).

Given that HIV is more abundant in male sperm than in vaginal secretions, and that women are eighteen times more likely to be infected by men then men by women, it is highly possible that many of these football players were infected prior to their alleged sex with "Lisa," the pseudonym the author uses to describe his acquaintance. Furthermore, the author has not considered the possibility that the young men whom "Lisa" is purported to have infected may have been infected by engaging in sex with one another, and that "Lisa" is actually a "front" for closeted gay/bisexual practices. The author has also not considered the possibility of injection steroid abuse, a not uncommon practice among college athletes.

To make matters worse, the author moves on to another female acquaintance, "who I'll call Jane, a Rutgers College sophomore, who enjoys her sexuality. This semester Jane got drunk one evening and decided to put herself at risk by exploring her libido with three guys who live on her floor. In the heat of passion, no one thought about using condoms" (15). Once again women's sexuality, not men's, is being framed as insatiable and destructive. Although the author suggests that all those involved failed to use condoms, it is crucial to stress that men wear condoms, not women. Even if "Jane" insisted that the three men wear condoms, she could not physically force them to do so. The writer, all in all, is unreliable, and one is left questioning: Is it a date rape he's writing about?

What stands out in this column is the age-old myth of woman as chaos, destruction, and source of infection. The undergraduate's narrative on AIDS awareness focuses entirely on women as conduits of infection and immoral behavior; the fact that it is easier for women to be infected by men, and that they are more likely to be raped by men, is ignored. Furthermore, the column offers no advice or examples on how these scenarios could have been handled differently; instead, it fuels the dangerous linkage between "bad" women's sexuality and death; it suggests that women's sexuality is itself the path of destruction for men. As in Hawthorne's "Lady Eleanor," women are the "angel of death."

Robin Gorna discusses the idea of the HIV-infected woman as "the angel of death" (xiv). For another example of women, HIV, and "revenge sex," see David France's misogynist article "A Dangerous Woman." For a different point of view, see Gary Allen Fine's analysis of HIV-positive women.

13. A different tack is taken by American writer Katherine Anne Porter in her novella "Pale Horse, Pale Rider." Here Porter addresses the denial and silence surrounding the great influenza epidemic of 1917, a "war" that occurred at the same time as World War I and killed more than 600,000 Americans (Krieg, 17). Porter, who was herself a victim of influenza during World War I, suggests that the epidemic was ignored despite the fact that more Americans died of influenza than in combat. Similarly, HIV/AIDS activists and advocates for people with AIDS often point out that the death toll due to AIDS has surpassed the death toll of the Vietnam War.

14. Joseph Cady addresses the issue of avoidance of death and AIDS in his entry on AIDS literature in *The Gay and Lesbian Literary Heritage*. Cady applies the critical categories of "immersive" and "counterimmersive" to a survey of AIDS literature produced by and for gay men. Using this terminology devised to gauge how gay male writers negotiate the "untouchable," "unspeakable" topic of AIDS, Cady analyzes the work of Tony Kushner, Paul Monette, Allen Barnett, and other well-known literary figures (in Summers, 16–20). Cady asserts that "counterimmersive" AIDS literature colludes with mainstream denial of the physical and cultural ravages of AIDS; "immersive" literature approaches the topic directly, without resorting to distancing or softening techniques such as camp, sardonic humor, supernatural occurrences, or irony. For example, Tony Kushner's acclaimed *Angels in America: A Gay Fantasia on National Themes* is taken to task for its counterimmersive stance on HIV. Not only does Kushner couch the topic of AIDS in supernatural elements and lengthy speeches on intellectual history, but his play makes the heterosexual marriage of Harper and Joe Pitt a major focus.

I agree with Cady that Kushner filters AIDS through the lens of the supernatural and the breakup of a heterosexual marriage, but I would argue that these methods of indirection have effects on cultural representations of women and AIDS as well. As in much AIDS literature and popular culture, Kushner's female characters are generated from dominant gender ideology. Thus, while Cady sees the figure of Harper Pitt as a symbol of Kushner's denial and "counterimmersiveness," I interpret this figure as representing how women's experiences in the epidemic are hidden behind the spectacle and domination of traditional gender; female characters are misused in an effort to destigmatize AIDS, to render mortality and queer sexuality less threatening.

15. For example, in a July 1997 letter to the *Irish Voice*, a reader says, "Having read two recent 'Dear Bridget' columns entitled 'AIDS: Is It Still a Threat?' and 'Surprise in the Blue Jeans,' I would like to ask a question—are there any young Irish women left today who believe in saving themselves for their wedding night?" (13). Significantly, the author (who identifies himself as Hugh Byrne of San Francisco, California) fails to direct his question to young Irish men.

16. As Susan Sontag argues, disease "is viewed as the occasion finally to behave well. At the least, the calamity of disease can clear the way for insight into lifelong self-deceptions and failures of character" (42).

17. For an example of women's resistance to traditional caretaking roles in relation to HIV, see Kimoto. Kimoto includes this revealing quote from one woman: "Are we supposed to take care of everyone all of the time? No way! It's about time that the community gets involved. And the community means men, women, and children!" (163). For more readings on HIV-positive women's experiences with caregiving, see Rudd and Taylor; Long and Ankrah.

18. As Linda Kerber argues, "One plausible way to read nineteenth-century defenses of separate spheres . . . is to single out the theme of breakdown . . ." (50). Similarly, Judith Williamson locates the theme of "breakdown" as central to many narratives on AIDS. As Kerber argues, "Surveys of history of political thought have shown that the habit of contrasting the 'worlds' of men and of women, the allocation of the public sector to men and the private sector (still under men's control) to women is older than western civilization" (47).

19. For example, Nancy Cott writes: "Idealization of woman as unfailingly virtuous, pious, and genteel left no room for cognizance of either her sensual nature or her physical needs for good health. The rhetorical direction of the cult of true womanhood was to spiritualize the female until she was almost literally 'disembodied.' Totally defined by her sex (reproduction), still the true woman was sexless (devoid of sexual passion)" (19).

20. As many contemporary feminist literary and cultural critics have argued, sentimentality is difficult to define because its meaning is contextual. Sentimental discourse is not an ancillary, ahistorical aesthetic category that one can banish or avoid. Rather, it is a deeply entrenched rhetoric with a complex history, within the realm of both the literary and the extraliterary. Sentimentality is confined neither to the literary text nor to the movie and television screen; rather, sentimental practices are a central frame structuring a wide range of cultural understandings and forms: medical research, political speeches, public policy, legal arguments, film, and popular literature.

The 1870s are typically declared the end of women's remarkable production of sentimental novels in the United States. Yet, as Laura Wexler proposes, long after the form waned in popularity, "sentimental ideology continued to mature in its power" (19). This was possible because the sentimental ideology encased in novels had "its concrete social institutionalization in schools, hospitals, prisons, and so on, whose building, staffing and operation quite naturally lag behind the literary imagination" (19).

Likewise, Gayle Pemberton analyzes sentimentality as a key determinant in local and national discussions of race relations between black and white women in the United States. In her essay "Hello, Stranger," she states, "What is so dispiriting about all this is that culturally we have not progressed beyond sentimentality—the default societally-induced emotional response—between strangers of different races" (281). Not only does Pemberton see sentimentality as a state ideology and practice that impedes complex debate; she uncovers its unfixed, chameleonlike quality: "sentimentality expresses itself in a variety of ways: arrogance, fear, hatred, curiosity and pity" (281).

Sentimental rhetoric wields considerable power in the creation of myths, metaphors, and images relating to many controversial social issues, including the sexual health crisis of AIDS.

For a discussion of sentimental rhetoric as a mediator of controversy, see Kathy E. Ferguson's treatment of sentimentality in the construction of contemporary Israeli national politics. Ferguson refers to the ideological production of the " 'meta-tear—the glue holding together a state-orchestrated collective identity" (95). For a discussion of sentimental rhetoric as the authority of emotion, see Catharine E. O'Connell, " 'The Magic of the Real Presence of Distress': Sentimentality and Competing Rhetorics of Authority."

21. See Jonathan Franzen's review of Russell Banks's novel *Bone*.

22. See Wexler.

23. See Walters.

24. Marcia Ian first suggested the term "immaculate infection" to me to describe representations of HIV-positive women and women with AIDS that rely on the image of innocent, female victims. Timothy Murphy also uses the term in his chapter "The Angry Death of Kimberly Bergalis" (89). I will discuss Murphy's use of the term and the case of Kimberly Bergalis in Chapter 2.

25. As Evelynn Hammonds suggests, the AIDS pandemic is "the great leveller of women" ("Seeing," 122).

26. For example, Hewitt points out that "privileged women [in the nineteenth century] were willing to wield their sex-specific influence in ways that, intentionally or unintentionally, exploited other women in the name of 'true womanhood' " (11).

27. See Adams for a discussion of how social and familial crises are used to exploit women psychologically and make women visible in problematic ways.

Chapter 2. Little Eva Revisited

1. See Golden, which explores the origins and lingering presence of the good woman as the one who sacrifices. Golden finds that in Western culture a true woman is a metaphoric (or actual) devotional mother who focuses on the pressing needs of family and community at the expense of her own needs. She argues that even women who have fought hard for accomplished, independent lives adhere to an updated version of the devotional mother icon.

2. Gun control emerged as an issue framed through the lens of the maternal. See Toner.

3. David Savran credits Joseph Roach with the suggestion that similarities exist between *Uncle Tom's Cabin* and *Angels in America*. See the first footnote in his essay.

4. Stowe addresses slavery in terms of "the separating of [heterosexual] families" and through the repeated assertion that white women's maternal culture is superior to the capitalistic, brutal world of (white) male politics and traffic in human bodies (*Uncle Tom's Cabin*, chap. 22). Stowe uses the figure of the good mother separated from her child as a powerful theme to produce sympathy in readers and foster social change. White women in Stowe's novel may not have much economic, political, or social power, but they have ample power as the morally and spiritually superior patriots devoted to saving America's Christian soul. Likewise, despite Kushner's transgender angel, he reinstalls conventional gender roles through the unambiguous female actor who plays the nurturing angel onstage, and through the characters of Harper Pitt and Hannah, Harper Pitt's Mormon mother-in-law. For instance, Harper Pitt is the ideal empath who intuits Prior Walter's feelings and fears of death even before he himself can articulate them. As David Savran puts it, "*Angels* seems to replicate many of the structures that historically have produced female subjectivity as Other. . . . And Hannah, despite her strength, is defined almost entirely by her relationship to her real son and to Prior, her surrogate son. Like Belize [the one black gay male character in the play], she is given the role of caretaker" (215).

Thus, caretaking, idealizations of feminine nurturance, and female sacrifice are underlying issues in *Angels in America*. Who should care for Prior Walter, the main character with AIDS, is a central conflict for Prior's errant lover, Louis Ironson. Through much of the play Louis expresses guilt over rejecting the role of caretaker, a role he equates with the good woman in Book I, where he delineates the ideal caretaker embodied in Mathilde, the selfless wife of the great William the Conqueror (51–52). Louis compares his personal and behavioral qualities with those of the ideal, devoted Mathilde, and realizes he cannot emulate her. He admits to himself and to other characters that he is afraid of disease, vomit, blood, wasting, and death. He even understands that he is a failure—"So what the fuck is the matter with me?"—yet his reluctance creates much of the poignancy of his character: he is neither noble nor exemplary (I:51–52).

Louis articulates the audience's selfishness, shame, and fear of physical suffering, death, and sacrifice, but the subtext is that Louis can never be the selfless figure that Western culture has conflated with the "ideal" woman. The other characters in the play, the women and the one character of color, Belize, take on these roles. Louis is the subject; he has too much sense of self, too much ego, too much of an identity to enact the paragon of utter devotion.

5. Cathy N. Davidson points out that "it is from [*Uncle Tom's Cabin*] more than any other, that the construct of the sentimental heroine was developed. The construct was based not on a woman character, but a young girl, Little Eva, whose angelic qualities doom her to an early, tear-wrenching death" (*Oxford Companion*, 787). Furthering the

idea that Little Eva symbolizes adult white womanhood, Hortense Spillers argues that Stowe "dispatches the child to do a woman's job; that is, the white woman's desire for the black man is displaced onto Little Eva" (44).

6. Timothy Murphy refers to this use of the respectable heterosexual woman as a "normalizing filter."

7. Also see pages 201–2, 264, 289, 294, 312–13.

8. For opposing views of Stowe's use of maternal discourse, see Roberson; Ammons.

9. For one of the most famous defenses of Stowe and Little Eva, see Tompkins. For a recent discussion of the novel's continued impact on American culture, see Berlant. Although Berlant does not focus on Little Eva per se, her idea that "the turn to sentimental rhetoric at moments of social anxiety constitutes a generic wish for an unconflicted world" (646) is particularly relevant to my analysis of sentimental AIDS.

10. See Stanovsky.

11. See Park and S. Harrington for fuller analyses of Bergalis's cultural work in terms of blame and saintly morality.

12. Hoffman adapts the pathos of the dying consumptive to fit a girl character with AIDS by emphasizing aspects of AIDS that most resemble tuberculosis: bodily wasting, weakness, and damaged, fragile lungs. For example, Amanda's father "can't allow himself to think about . . . the strain of each of her breaths, the rattling sound of each gasp" (205). Passages describing Amanda's pale face and skin, her wasting body, and her fevers resemble those that Stowe employs to describe the tubercular Little Eva: "Eva's little hands had grown thinner, and her skin more transparent, and her breath shorter; and . . . when she ran or played in the garden, as she once could for hours, she became soon tired and languid"; Eva has "a cough," a "feverent cheek . . . burning with hectic fever" (382–83).

13. As Nancy Cott explains, "The rhetorical direction of the cult of true womanhood was to spiritualize the female until she was almost literally disembodied" (19).

14. Hoffman's text clearly encourages us to read Laurel Smith as Amanda's adult self: Laurel "has long blond hair like Amanda's" (16); Polly notes that "Laurel Smith doesn't seem very much older than [Amanda]" (147). And when Ivan "walked into Laurel's cottage he realized it was exactly what Amanda would have chosen for herself" (179).

15. Nancy Cott observes that "Uncle Tom's Cabin amply demonstrates how the antislavery feelings of northern women gathered force from the image of slavery defiling the sacredness of the home, for both the black family and the white family" (16).

16. Dewey argues that "with Dickensian sensibility, Hoffman stage-manages Amanda's narrative. Unlike the mainstream victims of the disease, Amanda, by virtue of her age and the method by which she contracted the virus, can be accepted unambiguously by the reader as a victim. Thus Hoffman manages to elicit sentiment while neatly avoiding the tangling complexity of questions AIDS raises about love, sexuality, and death" (27). Dewey concludes that "At Risk is an uncomplicated exercise in the literature of doomed youth" (27). While Hoffman's fictional world is not equipped to deal with the paradoxes that characterize AIDS, the "tangle of complexity" that Dewey wants to be addressed does not seem to include the multiple ways in which HIV/AIDS impacts on women. For another essay on the politics of the innocent victim, see James Miller's "AIDS in the Novel: Getting it Straight" in his edited collection.

17. Eve Sedgwick argues: "If the obsessively homophobic focus of AIDS phobia . . . scapegoated gay men by (among other things) subjecting their sexual practice and lifestyles to a glaring and effectually punitive visibility, however, it worked

in an opposite way to regulate the visibility of most of the disease's other victims. So far, here, these victims have been among groups already most vulnerable—intravenous drug users, sex workers, wives and girlfriends of closeted men—on whom invisibility, or a public subsumption under the incongruous heading of gay men, can have no protective effect. . . . (It has been notable, for instance, that media coverage of prostitutes with AIDS has shown no interest in the health of the women themselves, but only in their potential for infecting men . . .)" (5–6). When Sedgwick refers here to the "intensive regulatory visibility" of gay men in AIDS discourse on the one hand and the "discursive erasure" of the disease's other victims on the other; and when she says that these "pairings are not only incommensurable . . . but very hard to interleave with each other conceptually," she unlocks one of the key arguments of this entire study. AIDS rhetoric, whether literary, critical, visual, or "popular," tends to render the idea of women with HIV infection or AIDS unspeakable. Women are routinely speakable in terms of traditional narratives: women as nurturers, social reformers, benevolent mothers, ministering angels, and people devastated by loss and mourning, but rarely as people at risk, rarely as people who are complex agents.

18. Pastore argues that Hoffman creates a character who experiences "the same prejudices" as other people with AIDS—gay men, IV drug users, inner city minorities (40). While Pastore eventually initiates a useful critique of the novel's apathy toward the inequalities of race and class differences, she nevertheless stands firm in her argument that Hoffman's text demonstrates how AIDS is a democratic disease.

Her analysis of gender in the novel can best be described as contradictory: she offers an analysis of Amanda's mother, Polly, as both a new feminist woman and a late 1980s version of the 1950s Donna Reed. For instance, Pastore explains Polly's erotic attraction to Ed Reardon as her only route to power: "As a doctor, Reardon . . . represents to Polly power she does not possess; as a woman, her only way of getting it is by attaching herself to a man who has it" (48). On a contrary note, Edith Milton argues that "[w]here [Hoffman] becomes pernicious is in her treatment of women" (17).

19. Critics also seem unconcerned with the novel's striking inability to imagine HIV infection in adult women. Joseph Cady points out that Hoffman places AIDS "in a situation that actually represents a minuscule proportion of the disease's epidemiology" ("Reaching," 239). However, my focus is less on the correspondence between AIDS epidemiology and the narrative than on how AIDS becomes an opportunity to revamp deeply conservative conceptions of gender and women, in particular, the idealization of women as nurturing angels. It is this insight that is often overlooked or trivialized in much AIDS theory, criticism, journalism, creative writing, and visual culture.

20. See Huston and Berridge.

21. I thank Gail Green-Anderson for pointing out how AIDS simultaneously renders women both not-women and the ultimate in womanhood.

22. It is notable that Fisher, who is Jewish and identifies as a Jew, was called a "Christmas angel."

23. Elizabeth Glaser's decision to be a stay-at-home mother meant that when AIDS came into her life the burden of dealing with childcare, medical care, and social ostracism fell largely on her. In reading her book, one is struck by how often her Hollywood husband is absent from the family's devastating ordeal.

24. Such a focus is the epitome of the ideal mother. Sacrificing self for children is so profoundly ingrained in our culture that anyone who even questions it is vulnerable to attack.

25. Glaser also includes photos of her family, but hers are not as staged as Fisher's. Glaser's photographs are more along the lines of home movies, while Fisher's resemble professional family photos.

26. It is important to note that Mary Fisher's children will most likely succumb to a fate far different from that of most AIDS orphans in the United States. Fisher was born into a prominent, wealthy, connected family. She is personal friends with such luminaries as Gerald and Betty Ford, George and Barbara Bush, and Larry Kramer, and she has access to the best mental and physical health care for herself and her sons.

27. Flavia Rando argues that the AIDS Memorial Quilt symbolically represents a feminine/maternal product that transforms deviant gay men into recognizable human beings. Seen from the perspective of the mourning mother, gay men are brought under "the cover of the quilt," where they experience lasting maternal care in death. Fisher's speech exemplifies this theme.

28. Perhaps the most remarkable example of repression of rage and anger appears in the testimony of another woman, Debbie Runions: "The question I am asked most often is, 'How do you feel about the man who transferred the virus to you?' My answer has changed over the year. When Luke did not return my call to tell me he had taken the test, I felt as though he had discarded me and my request as unimportant. I became concerned that he was knowingly spreading the virus to other unsuspecting women and putting their lives in danger. . . . My philosophy, however, is that we are all responsible for our own behavior. Although Luke was no doubt extremely infected with the virus, and he may indeed have known that he was infected, I was a grown woman who had heard about AIDS, knew what it took to protect myself, and did not. . . . Although my own personal ethics demand that I no longer engage in sexual intercourse, I do not hold Luke responsible for my infection. I give him the respect he deserves as one of the greatest teachers in my life. The disciplines I have learned through him have been extremely difficult—trials by fire" (70–71).

29. For an interesting discussion of celebrity mothers as instructors in mothering and morality, see Susan Douglas.

Chapter 3. Absent Mothers and Missing Children

1. The repeated appearance of the child in visual and print culture on AIDS to mediate moral judgment is noteworthy. In the film *Philadelphia* (1993) the main character with AIDS, Andrew Beckett, is visually redeemed when his sister encourages him to cradle her newborn baby. In *Boys on the Side* (1995), the dying heroine's deceased young brother makes a ghostly appearance and prepares his infected sister for the afterlife, a trope that evokes the suffering white woman who both defends the nation against moral corruption and teaches it compassionate democracy. (Both films are discussed in Chapter 4.) *A Place for Annie*, a made-for-television drama that I discuss in this chapter, is centered on a nine-week-old infant, Annie Marsten, who is born HIV positive to a drug-addicted mother. And a child with AIDS named Anika plays a crucial role in mediating the stigma of AIDS in the 1995 novel *touch* (see Chapter 5). As discussed in Chapter 2, *Uncle Tom's Cabin* repeatedly evokes dead children, culminating in the spectacular death of Little Eva, and Hoffman's *At Risk* reworks this tradition around the death of a child, Amanda Farrell, as does the film *Boys on the Side*.

2. I am grateful to John Nguyet Erni for this concise phrase.

3. I agree with Keniston's assessment, but not because I think American society truly values the individual lives of privileged white girls. The realities of incest, childhood sexual abuse, eating disorders, and educational abuse, which affect even girls of

privileged populations, suggest exploitation rather than genuine humanity. The point is that white girlhood and womanhood have been historically used to control what counts as an American citizen; AIDS-infected queers and drug users are often placed outside the nation.

4. Harriet Beecher Stowe's text is literally put on "trial" in Robert Alexander's 1996 play *I Ain't Yo' Uncle*. Alexander focuses on the distortions of African American life and history created by Stowe's novel and "rewrites" the famous antislavery narrative. Organized around bringing Harriet Beecher Stowe to trial for, as Alexander's Topsy puts it, "creatin' stereotypes," the play opens with the characters of George, Eliza, Topsy, and Tom presenting their individual reasons for dissatisfaction. The remainder of the play is composed of each character's own revision of the action and dialogue.

For example, at the end of the play, the character Harriet Beecher Stowe tries to talk back to the characters, and George tells her: "Harriet, could you sit down and be quiet? This ain't about you anymore. It's about us writing our stories" (89). Even more pertinent to my discussion here are the agency and anger Alexander provides Topsy: "Stop calling me monkey! I guess you're still wondering how Goldilocks [Eva] got sick all of a sudden. . . . I guess it never crossed your mind a little monkey like me had anything to do wid it" (67). To Alexander, *Uncle Tom's Cabin* is a cultural bridge that links nineteenth-century racial stereotypes and injustice to late-twentieth-century forms of stereotyping and injustice.

5. Abolitionist writers such as Stowe did not see African Americans as equals in the legal and social sense. White superiority suffused everything that Stowe accomplished and argued for, and *Uncle Tom's Cabin* is a good example of her conflicted and confused views. Stowe used sentimental domesticity and Christianity to frame her arguments, with a special emphasis on the separation of mother and child as a breach of nature, but the novel did little to bring about "social justice and the promotion of racial equality" (Nuernberg, 269). Idealizing blacks in fiction but making clear that "they are not high enough to be part of society" preserved the idea of whiteness as the standard and the norm (Nuernberg, 269).

Stowe assiduously highlighted the depravity of slavery for whites and blacks and suggested that ending slavery was the only way to achieve white salvation (Ducksworth, 205). Christian values compelled Stowe to argue for the protection of black women's virtue and roles as mothers and for the view that blacks had souls. Patricia Turner points out that "Stowe set out to write a corrective, a story that might mitigate some of the damage being inflicted by her Southern contemporaries. Because of her own upbringing and experiences, she too was a culprit in the perpetuation of a Eurocentric worldview. She grew up in a society that privileged white over black in subtle and unsubtle ways. At the same time that she was struggling to undo some of the grosser forms of racism, her sense of white superiority infused her words" (67).

Stowe's Uncle Tom functions as an exceptional literary hero: he is brave and strong, but not in a threatening way; he is a moral and spiritual figure who sacrifices himself for his family and community. As a good Christian, Uncle Tom never lies, cheats, steals, drinks, or disobeys his master and mistress. Uncle Tom may be too good to be true, but he is a genuine Christian hero. This character aided Stowe in achieving the political goal of persuading white readers to end slavery. But neither she, nor her famous abolitionist novel, nor her other abolitionist rhetoric dismantled the social institution of white superiority. Stowe believed that every person deserved freedom from bondage and the opportunity to create a Christian-centered heterosexual family, but these beliefs did not alter the pervasive underlying cultural assumption that white people were superior.

Her characterizations of Aunt Chole and Topsy similarly indicate her moral, Christian commitment to introducing representations of black women and girls into the national consciousness. But these characters ultimately solidify racial myths of black women and girls. Aunt Chole consolidates the view of black woman as the desexed mammy, the happy nurturer and server, and Topsy, as I have been arguing, is the prototype of the pickaninny, the mischievous entertainer, complete with baggy clothes and toothy grin. As David Levy points out, "Those who attacked slavery in fiction portrayed the races in precisely the same terms as those who defended it" (quoted in Carby, 33). Lisa Watt MacFarlene suggests that critics must analyze how "Stowe's sentimentalism . . . presented the white experience as normative; Stowe's abolitionism was radical in its demand for emancipation, but it relied upon racist assumptions of difference" (857).

6. The term "postsentimental" is Berlant's: "An author's text's refusal to reproduce the sublimation of subaltern struggles into conventions of narrative satisfaction and redemptive fantasy might be called 'postsentimentality,' a resistant strain of the sentimental domain" (655).

7. "Postsentimental narratives are lacerated by ambivalence" (Berlant, 655).

8. In *Baby Doctor*, Klass does not explicitly refer to the racial aspects of sentimentality, as she does in her novel. Instead, she writes about the inevitability of sentimentality when the subject is an ill child: "The problem with writing about sick children is that it is virtually impossible to escape sentimentality. Take a picture of a child, any child, and the odds are reasonably good that the picture will be cute; that's how thousands of parents generate millions of adorable pictures. Write in the caption, this child is dying of AIDS (or cancer or whatever), and you immediately have a tug at the heartstrings. Articles about pediatric AIDS, TV movies, magazine cover stories, all tend inexorably toward such phrases as 'innocent victims.' They are appealing, they are adorable, and they are dying. With adult AIDS victims there is a profound tendency to attach blame, to identify the risk factor and to point the finger. . . . And with children, of course, no one, however self-righteous, however eager to blame the victim, can claim that dubious high moral ground. Children, whatever their diseases, remain quintessentially innocent, and of course, adorable" (196–97).

9. As I discuss in this chapter, media reports and medical research fuel and reproduce the cult of sacrificial woman, even though such a stance is dangerous to women's health. Statements such as "I focused on my child. I knew I had to find him an AIDS doctor so I started with that. I didn't even think about seeking care for myself" are considered moving and evidence of mother love (Ladonna, "Listen to Children," 1). This kind of sacrificial discourse fuels the invisibility of women's bodies by focusing on women as vessels that bring infected babies to the medical field and to society.

10. At the 12th World Conference on AIDS, Rebecca Denison states: "There was almost nothing about getting men to take responsibility for condom use with their female partners, even though men control when and how a couple has sex in most cultures" ("Pregnancy and Perinatal Transmission," 6).

11. I am basing my discussion of the creation of the welfare state on Gwendolyn Mink's "The Lady and the Tramp: Gender, Race and the Origins of the American Welfare State." For articles on the dismantling of AFDC in the 1990s, see Bojar; Deprez; Kahn et al.; McCallum; and Tobin.

12. See Paula Martinac's article on the 1998 Supreme Court decision in *Bragdon v. Abbott*. Martinac looks at some of the underlying assumptions of this decision, such as the idea that HIV-positive pregnant women are not "mommy material."

13. See Farber for a fuller discussion of this issue as well as other issues related to HIV and pregnancy. Ironically, Farber's essay does not explore how the fusing of

women and children downplays the mother's health. However, Farber does include a chilling excerpt from an internal memo on the 076–trial, the AZT pregnancy trial: "Although safety [is] unknown it can be argued that any possibility of stopping transmission to the fetus outweighs perceived risks to the woman" (quoted in Farber, 57).

14. See Hansen.

15. A good example of indifference toward American babies whose mothers belong to the economically and socially created ranks of the young and poor is the recent New York State court case involving the death of Tabitha Walrond's infant son, Tyler. Tabitha Walrond was convicted of criminal negligence because she experienced difficulties breast-feeding her infant and he died. When she sought medical care for Tyler at the Medicaid HMO in New York City, she was turned away because the infant's Medicaid card had not yet arrived. According to E. Frances White, "City contracts with Medicaid HMOs, including HIP, require them to see infants, whether they have a card or not. The card arrived in the mail weeks after the infant's death." One of the jurors who found Tabitha Walrond guilty said, "She was failed, but she should have been strong enough to do more" (quoted in White, "HMO Kills Baby").

Walrond's case has garnered the attention of several feminist organizations, such as the New York City Black Radical Congress Feminist Caucus, the National Black Radical Congress, and the New York chapter of the National Organization of Women. Activists point out that Walrond is being blamed for being poor, young, black, unmarried, and a mother. White motherhood and domesticity rely upon enormous economic and social resources, and Walrond belongs to a group of young women demonized for not reflecting the normative, white, married, heterosexual ideal. In a sense, Walrond is being blamed for exposing the impossibility of idealized motherhood for most young women.

Chapter 4. The Lesbian Mammy

1. Donald Bogle's film history *Toms, Coons, Mulattoes, Mammies and Bucks: An Interpretive History of Blacks in American Films* is considered a primary text in film studies and history, as well as in African American studies. However, some postmodern film theorists might find Bogle's method of focusing on "stereotypes" and "images" of black people in film outdated. For example, Ellis Hanson's *Outtakes: Essays on Queer Theory and Film* critiques the stereotypes and the politics of representation method as theoretically naive and oversimplified.

However, as Suzanna Walters contends, although pre-poststructuralist criticism of "stereotypes" and "images" criticism is theoretically unsophisticated and naive, the advantage of a stereotype/images approach—in contrast to the language-focused, "signification" work on representation celebrated today—is that it forcefully stresses historical and political context. Although Hanson would disagree with Walters's assessment, Walters points out that "signification" theorists often fail to consider the social realities of people's lives, an aspect that was also foregrounded in the seventies' "images of women," or stereotypes of women, work.

2. Feminist critic Patricia Hill Collins has considerable insight into characters such as Blanche White: "For reasons of economic survival, African-American women may play the mammy role in paid work settings. But within African-American communities these same women often teach their own children something quite different" ("Mammies," 73). For further insight into the social construction of black women as mammies, see Collins, "Mammies." For a discussion of images of black women as mammies in literature, see Harris, especially chapter 7. For an example of how the in-

vention of the mammy continues to exert influence in contemporary popular culture, see Manring.

3. Negotiating the terrain of black women's bodies, sexualities, and identities in terms of white women's tears has a long history in American culture. In mid-nineteenth-century America, the writer Harriet Jacobs wrote of the mass rape of black women and girls by their white slavemasters in her book *Incidents in the Life of a Slave Girl*. Jacobs strategically filtered her own experiences as a female slave through the rhetoric and conventions of "white" literary sentimentality. A central trope Jacobs employed was the "good white mother." In this way, she was able to appease white middle-class women of the North, gain entry into the white-controlled world of publishing, and encourage abolitionist activity. Jacobs's use of sentimentality as a language to signal black women's experiences is often strained, and yet this "straining" conveys incongruous doubled meanings that capture the racial politics, as well as the racial subtext, of literary sentimentality.

In one passage of her book, Jacobs directly exposes the politics of white women's tears. In chapter 28, "Aunt Nancy," Jacobs recounts how her aunt was worked to death by Mrs. Flint; yet when Aunt Nancy finally died from years of abuse, Mrs. Flint "became very sentimental" and demanded that Nancy be interred in the white people's burial ground (146).

Jacobs's writing and Neely's character, in the context of women, AIDS, and representation, suggest the political effect of representations of white women's tears on black women's lives. In general, African American women are typically construed in AIDS reportage, popular culture, and medical and scientific discourse as promiscuous drug abusers who infect innocent children and men. Critics explain that these "roles" for black women precede AIDS, and can be found in representations of women in a wide variety of public health campaigns and documents throughout the twentieth century. Despite some social and legal gains produced by black civil rights and women's liberation, images of African American women in popular culture and public policy debates continue to fuel historically ingrained "roles" for black women.

Evelynn Hammonds's work on race, gender, AIDS, the media, and medical history addresses the roles of race and gender in AIDS. Also see Juhasz.

4. Critics, artists, and writers question the critique of the mammy stereotype as a method of analysis of black women and representation. Hilton Als has been exploring the "Mammy" and "Negress" in a way that seems to move beyond positions such as McCaskill and Phillips's, who insist that representations of African American womanhood continue to "revolve around reductive roles of mammy or whore" (121). Rather than discount the ubiquitous mammy paradigm that permeates literature and popular culture, Als approaches it as a site of representation's own undoing, where black women's spectatorship and complex responses to media images suggest a subjectivity that shrewdly filters out racist values central to mainstream representation and culture. This rich work on representation and the mammy is compelling and creative, but I wonder how relevant Als's standpoint is to the work of identifying the material politics of representations of black women and AIDS.

5. For an interesting discussion of how the dominant culture exploits a group's symbolic usefulness, see Vaidhyanathan.

6. A view of the Hollywood film opposite from the one presented here is Ellis Hanson's *Outtakes: Essays on Queer Theory and Film*. Hanson writes that "Hollywood, despite its history of censorship and its pretense to heterocentrism, is one of the queerest institutions ever invented" (7). Not all artists agree. As reported in a recent article in *Ms. Magazine*, film producers have approached Barbara Neely about her Blanche White mystery series. Neely says she fears that a screen version of her character

would result in "an Aunt Jemima, or someone lighter, thinner, younger, and cuter" (79). She has refused all offers to use her character, and she has refused the offer of writing her own screenplay based on her character.

7. This, of course, is not the case in contemporary fiction, where black women writers have created—and continue to create—fiction that explores the lives and struggles of working-class African American women. A few pioneering examples include Mary Helen Washington's collection *Black-Eyed Susans: Classic Stories by and about Black Women*, Toni Morrison's *Sula* and *Beloved*, and Alice Walker's *The Color Purple*. Also, a film such as *The Color Purple* offers, however mediated, points of identification, connection, and alternative readings for black women viewers.

8. I am using Valerie Smith's concept, to "mean less or mean differently" (9). Hazel Carby argues that the typical nineteenth-century sentimental plot involves a white, privileged female character who gets to die a lavish sentimental death, while the black female character, who survives her numerous violations and mistreatment, is deemed less womanly for doing so. As Carby states, the black woman's ability to endure slavery, rape, and the humiliation of servitude renders her ineligible for the ranks of true womanhood—"the true heroine would rather die than be sexually abused" (34). This racialized sentimental legacy, also known as the "cult of true womanhood," is alive and well in cultural and artistic work on AIDS.

9. As Patricia Hill Collins explains, "Even though [the mammy] may be well loved and may wield considerable authority in her white 'family,' the mammy still knows her 'place' as obedient servant" ("Mammies," 71).

10. See V. Smith, 8.

11. Goldberg has also played a Space Age mammy on television, on *Star Trek: The Next Generation*. "The character of Guinan, who seems to have existed for centuries and in several dimensions, is the ship's bartender. And, while she does not have the official rank of ship's 'counselor' (another female, a white, bosomy member of an 'empathic' species, is ship therapist and basically points out the obvious), Guinan does provide insight all the time in the manner of a guru; she never has romantic or sexual liaisons; and is the Captain's special friend, giving him sage advice, protecting him, looking out for him. Also, Guinan's race has enslavement in its past" (Ian).

12. Admittedly, Janet Maslin and Elizabeth Pincus are "popular" as opposed to "academic" critics, yet their views and silences often resemble the views and silences found in academic cultural criticism. Furthermore, academic criticism on such themes as lesbian and gay studies, AIDS, black women, representation, and feminism does not occur in a cultural vacuum, despite the cherished image of the ivory tower removed from the world. For example, Evelynn Hammonds's work exposes the erasure of black women's sexualities and lives in popular as well as academic discourses on AIDS.

13. *Thelma and Louise* is a far more complex film of popular feminism than either *Boys on the Side* or *Terms of Endearment*. *Terms of Endearment*, similar to many film and fictional treatments of AIDS, uses the occasion of a white dying mother as a springboard for antifeminist backlash and mandatory gendered caretaking. *Thelma and Louise*, by contrast, shocked cultural commentators, resulting in widespread condemnation and debate about the film. For a good summary of the debate surrounding *Thelma and Louise*, see Walters, 1–28.

14. Contrast Maslin's discussion of Goldberg's portrayal of Jane as an "outsider" to Patricia Hill Collins's views on African American women as strangers in their own land: "The status of African-American women as outsiders or strangers becomes the point from which other groups define normality. . . . As the 'Other' of society who can never really belong, strangers threaten the moral and social order. But they are si-

multaneously essential for its survival because those individuals who stand at the margins of society clarify its boundaries. African-American women, by not belonging, emphasize the significance of belonging" ("Mammies," 68). Collins goes on to explain that African American women's "outsider" status often provides them with a powerful, critical point of view that allows them to dismantle conventional and dominant ways of thinking. Yet for Maslin, the meaning of Goldberg's—and Jane's—outsiderness is both mundane and mysterious.

15. As Hammonds argues, from "the production of the image of a pathologized black female 'other' in the eighteenth century" to the myth of the "loose," hypersexual black female that was produced during and after slavery and Reconstruction, representations of black women's sexualities have been fraught with silence, unease, and racist mythologies ("Black," 132–33).

One strategy developed by late-nineteenth-century and early-twentieth-century black women social reformers was to counter the myth of the black woman as the "embodiment of sex" with the image of black women as the embodiment of supermorality—an image that still has a far-reaching impact on contemporary representations of black women, as Donald Bogle's history of black actors in film suggests (Hammonds, "Black," 133). I discuss this history in more detail in the next chapter.

16. See Manring, 149–83.

17. While white female caretaking is often presented in AIDS discourse as involving HIV-negative and HIV-positive women whose love and tenderness rescue the stigmatized gay male from the realm of total abjection, no one performs this function for HIV-infected poor women or women of color on a representational level. The white middle-class female character may even possess a nonconventional trait, such as the imaginative, eccentric, drug-addicted Harper Pitt of Tony Kushner's *Angels in America*, or the funky lesbian helpmates in Paul Monette's novel *Halfway Home* and Nisa Donnelly's *The Love Songs of Phoenix Bay*; but these female characters are nevertheless constructed in terms of the traditional idea of the good woman as the woman who cares. They act as "white" mammies, but because of their class and race privilege they are more often constructed as slim, ethereal "ministering angels" rather than as the sentimentalized figure of the hefty, black mammy. However, women of all races, classes, ages, and religions grapple with the construction of "bad" women or "good" women in AIDS discourse. Good women function as didactic role models to a heartless AIDS-phobic society; bad women shore up the division between those who deserve sympathy and services and those who do not. Rarely are complex women located in diverse communities where they struggle with homophobia, racism, and sexism as well as with HIV. Even when a woman herself is HIV positive, women's actual experiences in the epidemic are often treated as peripheral and incidental.

18. For a discussion of fake visibility, see Schulman, in particular, "Conclusion: The Creation of a Fake Public Homosexuality."

19. Evelynn Hammonds observes of representation in the AIDS epidemic that "black women are victims that are once again the 'other' of the 'other,' the deviants of the deviants, regardless of their sexual identities and practices" ("Black," 141).

20. Emotional white femininity in sentimental novels is addressed in Danica. Danica offers an example of how white sentimental glorification (also) masks class politics and childhood sexual abuse: "I push myself to read harder books. Nothing gives me a hint of a life like mine. Nothing is even close. There are saints, there are Alcott's *Little Women* and there are holy martyrs. There is nothing else. I am wrong" (19–20). Similarly, Dorothy Allison's *Bastard Out of Carolina*, described by one reviewer as "one of those unusual books that show childhood abuse without sentimentality or simplicity," reveals class politics embedded in sentimental narrative.

21. Through its mainstreaming, *Boys on the Side*, similar to *Touched by an Angel*, may offer affirmation to some people with AIDS; but this fact does not rule out critical analysis.

22. "A film may have incredibly revolutionary standpoints merged with conservative ones" (hooks, *Reel*, 3). I think multiple and contradictory standpoints are prevalent in films on AIDS.

23. Similar uses of the supernatural are found in Tony Kushner's *Angels in America—Part One: Millennium Approaches*.

24. In her work on women's sensation novels, Ann Cvetkovich argues that the difficulty with the lavish emotional display of suffering in these texts is not that it expresses so-called manipulative, "feminine" culture (a patriarchal view) or that it provides women readers with the opportunity for fantasy, identification, and potential empowerment (a literary feminist view). Rather, the problem lies in the "political consequences of the construction of the figure of the suffering woman" (98). Sentimental novels potentially empower female readers by urging them to recognize how patriarchal culture represses women's pain, but they also suggest that the expression of feeling is in itself the way to alleviate the conditions of oppression—"relief would be if she could only articulate her feelings" (Cvetkovich, 98). By contrast, relief for Neely's Blanche White does not occur when her boss, Grace, articulates her feelings. In fact, Blanche experiences Grace's articulation of her feelings as one more instance of exploitation. Blanche's unraveling of the politics of the suffering white woman supports Cvetkovich's argument that the privileging of emotional articulation alone "cast[s] social problems as emotional ones in order to construct emotional solutions" when, in fact, the solutions most desperately needed are economic, social, and political reform (131).

25. In James Baldwin's essay "Everybody's Protest Novel," he blasts the kind of sentimentality that we see infused throughout *Boys on the Side*. To Baldwin, sentimentality is the snuffing out of "true" emotion. Rather than a language of genuine feelings, Baldwin sees sentimentality as a process of dehumanization and characterizes it as "the mark of dishonesty, the inability to feel" (14). He says that "the wet eyes of the sentimentalist betray his aversion to experience, his fear of life, his arid heart; and it is always, therefore, the signal of secret and violent inhumanity, the mask of cruelty" (14). As Hazel Carby has shown, scores of black female characters have been dehumanized, made invisible, and belittled in white women's sentimental literature. Again, Blanche White's critique of white women's "Mammy-save-me eyes" brings to mind what Laura Wexler calls "tender violence"(9–38): each time her self-absorbed employer breaks into tears, Blanche's invisibility and oppression are intensified.

26. As Helen Taylor points out, some feminists have consistently celebrated the novel and film in terms of Scarlett O'Hara's determination and leadership, while black feminists "are left to point to the political problems" (114). Taylor explains that white feminist celebration would require "both turning a blind eye to [the novel's and film's] white supremacist southern propaganda, and entering into an unholy alliance with the crudest southern chauvinism and the activities of the Ku Klux Klan" (115). Simply put, what some feminist critics and readers interpret as women's resistance to domination, other feminist critics and readers interpret as reactionary racial stereotypes and class ideology. This tension within a white, middle-class, feminist sensibility that challenges patriarchal dominance yet capitulates to reductive constructions of racial, economic, and sexual inequalities and identities has been vigorously exposed by numerous critics, including bell hooks, Audre Lorde, Hazel Carby, Patricia Hill Collins, and Barbara Smith, to name just a few. Barbara McCaskill and Layli Phillips

assert, "We're downright weary of our typecast roles as the laughable Topsies of women's lib or the Beulahs who breast-feed the feminist imagination" (117).

27. For an excellent discussion of how Hollywood uses myths about black male sexuality in a similar way, see Tania Modleski's analysis of *The Green Mile* in "In Hollywood, Racist Stereotypes Still Earn Oscar Nominations." Although Modleski does not touch on this, I would also argue that *The Green Mile* offers a deformed view of health care in the main black character's excessive, Christ-like self-sacrifice coupled with his mysterious healing powers. In this way, John Coffey resembles the black mammy.

Chapter 5. What Looks Like Progress

1. See Patricia Hill Collins, *Black Feminist Thought: Knowledge, Consciousness, and the Politics of Empowerment.*

2. On this point Virginia Valian argues, "The act of physical nurturance is extrapolated to the personality realm, so that we—both men and women—see women not only as literally nurturing but also as metaphorically nurturing" (116).

3. Both Valian and Golden explore metaphoric mothering, but Golden also focuses on the connections between sacrifice and race.

4. Barbara Ogur warns that statistics and epidemiology tell us only where the virus has been, not necessarily who is being infected now or who will be infected in the future: "[W]e must be very cautious about what conclusions we draw from epidemiology. The most consistent data are from the CDC, categorized by ethnicity, age, and by simplified risk behaviors. These data still show the majority of cases of AIDS in men who have had sex with men or in people who have used injecting drugs; it shows that the majority of U.S. women with AIDS are African American and Hispanic. However, since it takes eight to ten years for AIDS to develop after infection with HIV, these data are simply a reflection of where the virus was eight to ten years ago, a fossilized footprint" (150).

Likewise, Gena Corea reports that women who look at representations of AIDS and don't see themselves are shocked when they test positive. For example, referring to Penny Abernathy's story, Corea writes: "In those television specials, the people with AIDS had been almost all gay men. She had never seen a woman with AIDS on television. Now, she, a woman, was infected!" (75). Women also report that they are repeatedly refused HIV tests when they ask for them. Corea documents a case in which a woman repeatedly asked to be tested but her doctor refused. The woman, not surprisingly, went on to develop AIDS (166).

5. For a discussion of how current black activists and leaders are responding to and grappling with the connections among racism, sexism, homophobia, and heterosexism, see Cohen. Also see Cohen and Jones; Ards.

6. In May 1998 the Congressional Black Caucus called for a Public Health Emergency on HIV/AIDS. See Maldonado.

7. For an excellent article on AIDS and the black church, see Blaxton.

8. Kristal Brent Zook points out, "For all of the club movement's good works, including employment agencies and self-improvement programs for women, it never abandoned its need to play it safe and be polite" (88).

9. Also in 1997, Carolyn Ferrel's "Don't Erase Me," a short story about a fourteen-year-old girl with HIV infection, appeared in the author's critically acclaimed collection *Don't Erase Me: Stories.*

10. Women's diaries, journals, and letters have a long history in American literature. They are a rich source of information for writers, historians, and literary schol-

ars. Feminist scholarship on diaries and letters has contributed to an expanded understanding of how historical and literary knowledge is produced, and contemporary women writers continue to experiment with these forms.

These forms address diverse themes, ranging from frontier life to highly self-reflexive, psychological examinations of everything from heterosexual marriage to breast cancer. Letters and diaries also provide women the opportunity to respond to their marginalization in the dominant culture by critiquing patriarchal attacks with alternative perspectives and understandings. As a literary form, this work expresses the writer's desire to transform the ephemeral nature of everyday life into a permanent aesthetic form and to communicate with other women.

11. A reader who attended one of Cleage's readings reported in an on-line discussion that Cleage told him, "One of the writers that has been a contemporary influence on me has been Alice Walker . . . because she is brave enough to write about anything—fearless. When I have my reservations about writing about something, I ask myself, 'What would Alice do' and then I proceed to write."

12. "And afterwards, when I could make myself talk again, I crawled to the telephone and placed two long-distance calls: there was nobody local who would care" (13). I do not know the area of Long Island where Jordan was living, but whenever I read this sentence I wonder if there was a rape crisis center she could have contacted.

13. A complex representation of black female identity, motherhood, and communal care is Toni Morrison's *Beloved*—"Unless carefree, motherlove was a killer" (132). Morrison's *Beloved* offers an astonishing narrative on black motherhood and female identity in the context of crisis. When Sethe cries out that Beloved was her "best thing," Paul D. replies, "You your best thing, Sethe. You are" (272–73).

14. Theodore's brother, a gay man who died of AIDS, was shunned by his family and died alone. This is why Theodore studies public health and has contacts with AIDS organizations. My argument is not with community service per se, but with community service that submerges Rayna's identity as an artist.

15. Patricia Hill Collins might argue that changes in Rayna's behavior symbolize "rejection of separateness and individual interest as the basis of either community organization or individual self-actualization. Instead, the connectedness with others and common interest expressed by community othermothers models a very different value system, one whereby Afrocentric feminist ethics of caring and personal accountability move communities forward" ("Black Women," 207). Thus, from Collins's perspective, "the importance that people of African descent place on mothering" explains the changes in a character such as Rayna ("Black Women," 198).

But there is a danger in promoting a romanticized view of women of African descent in relation to mothering. Lynde Francis, an HIV-positive African woman, who spoke about breast-feeding at the 1998 World Conference on AIDS in Geneva, offers a view of African women as mothers that is missing in the communal paradigm: "While I feel strongly about the rights of all women to reproductive health choices, I represent a continent where the majority have no choice, voice or ownership in or of their reproduction. Millions are literally owned by their families and viewed as marketable sources of babies. They are defined by their fecundity, devalued and often discarded if they fail to produce" (5). Patrice DiQuinzio writes, "Despite Collins's warning about the effects of the stereotype of the strong, suffering black mother, her account of black mothers and daughters cannot entirely resist this vision" (228).

16. Research on HIV and incest indicates that there are indirect and direct links between sexual assault and HIV infection in women and girls. The indirect connection is that the coping strategies of survivors of childhood sexual abuse set them up for increased exposure to HIV infection. For example, one prevalent response to childhood

sexual abuse is to withdraw, but an equally common response is to recreate sexual encounters in which survivors assume the passive, silenced role that they experienced when they were sexually abused. Another common reaction of survivors of childhood sexual abuse is to engage in alcohol and drug use. Third, survivors of childhood sexual abuse are more likely to work as sex workers than people who were not abused as children. Thus, childhood sexual abuse increases HIV-related risk behaviors, increasing the chance of HIV infection.

Sexual assault and HIV in girls are directly linked when HIV is transmitted during sexual violence, as dramatized in Sapphire's novel. Precious Jones contracts HIV as a result of the repeated incest-rape committed by her biological father, who is HIV positive and eventually dies of AIDS. Precious writes in her journal that the first instance of incest occurred when she was still wearing diapers. According to the U.S. National Victim Center, 29 percent of all rapes occur when the child is under eleven years old (quoted in Vassall, 3). In addition, Sapphire claims that "[a]lmost fifty percent [of teen pregnancies] are the result of much older people and parents abusing them in the home" (Fitzpatrick, 36).

The response from AIDS leaders and organizations to the link between HIV infection and sexual assault is denial. According to the Centers for Disease Control, there are only "28 *documented* cases of HIV infection through child sexual assault" (Vassall, 3). However, while 500,000 cases of sexual assault are reported each year, "an estimated 1,500,000 more are not reported" (quoted in Vassall, 3). E. Rikki Vassall writes that "the overlap between high incidences of HIV infection [in young women] (ages 15–25) and high incidences of rape (ages 16–24) is frightening" (3). According to Esma Polkinghorne, the still prevailing conception of AIDS as a male disease, combined with the image of incest and sexual abuse as women's issues, explains why researchers are reluctant to investigate the connection. As a result, the tracking and documentation of HIV infection via sexual assault are simply not happening.

17. I think Sapphire is also fictionalizing the deadly impact of heterosexism on black heterosexuals. For an in-depth discussion of heterosexism as a central oppression in all black people's lives, not just in queer people's lives, see Cohen and Jones.

18. Cathy Cohen and Tamara Jones argue that "young black women learn that the development of their individual characters, intellect, and independent strength must at all times be secondary to their dependence and obedience to black men" (93).

19. This same defiance is brilliantly evident in the frontispiece to *A Positive Life: Portraits of Women Living with HIV,* which portrays a photograph of an HIV-positive African American woman wearing a white wedding dress and veil.

20. Cleage frames Joyce's service in terms of sixties activism, but it is important to note the difference between service and political activism. In a recent on-line discussion on a women's studies listserv, Beatrice Kachuck notes the difference. Service involves helping "people solve a problem within an existing structure or system. . . . Activism, on the other hand, is work that tries to change a structure or system, e.g., analyze conditions that lead to illiteracy, hunger and battering of women. Either could be paid or unpaid."

21. There is a striking contradiction in Cleage's presentation of the character Eddie. Cleage has Eddie announce that he is planning to murder Tyrone and Frank, two teenage boys who are on the wrong path, as his way of protecting his family: Ava, Joyce, and Imani. Like Sapphire, Cleage seems to want to introduce questions about revenge when the perpetrators are black instead of white, but her handling of this explosive issue is confusing at best and reactionary at worst.

22. They each exploit what Virginia Valian sees as a culturally induced difference between men and women: "What finally enmeshes women in their inequitable situa-

tion is the real joy to be gained from exercising their duty, a pleasure most men have not developed a taste for" (44).

23. As Lillian Faderman puts it, "The abstract category 'woman' to which all females have been taught they belong is still belittled and stigmatized in almost all cultures, and that stigmatization has awful effects on females, whether or not those females agree that 'woman' really exists. . . . Strategic essentialism as applied to feminism begins by acknowledging difference between females, but also acknowledges the need to band together under the banner 'woman' wherever such banding can be mutually helpful to females" (Afterword, 228).

Chapter 6. Conclusion

1. In reading Als's description of the good Negress in literature, I am struck by the similarities between this figure and the "good woman" in AIDS discourse: "Given the written material in which she [the Negress] appears, it is difficult to feel one is in the presence of a person; by extension, it is difficult to imagine her making an appearance in literature as anything other than a tiresome colored woman, weeping over her attempts to be a good neighbor" (47).

2. See Barbara Bates's study of African Americans and tuberculosis. "Bates notes that despite the fact that large numbers had the disease 'hospitals and sanatoriums often excluded blacks, and neither money nor personal recommendations could assure them acceptable care' " (quoted in Rothman, 260 n. 10).

WORKS CITED

I. Primary Sources

Alcott, Louisa May. *Little Women*. New York: Signet, 1983.
Alexander, Robert. "I Ain't Yo' Uncle." In *Colored Contradictions: An Anthology of Contemporary African-American Plays*, ed. Harry J. Elam Jr. and Robert Alexander. New York: Plume, 1996.
Allison, Dorothy. *Bastard Out of Carolina*. New York: Dutton, 1992.
Baldwin, James. "Everybody's Protest Novel." *Notes of a Native Son*. Boston: Beacon, 1955. 13–23.
Barnett, Allen. *The Body and Its Dangers*. New York: St. Martin's, 1990.
Boys on the Side. Dir. Herbert Ross. Perf. Whoopi Goldberg, Mary-Louise Parker, Drew Barrymore, Matthew McConaughey, Anita Gillette, James Remar, Amy Aquino, Dennis Boutsikaris, and Estelle Parsons. Warner Brothers, 1995.
Brown, Charles Brockden. *Arthur Mervyn, or, Memoirs of the Year 1793*. 1799–1800. Kent, Ohio: Kent State University Press, 1977.
Cleage, Pearl. *What Looks Like Crazy on an Ordinary Day*. New York: Avon Books, 1997.
Donnelly, Nisa. *The Love Songs of Phoenix Bay*. New York: St. Martin's, 1994.
Dowd, Maureen. "Proud Mary." *POZ*, October–November 1994, 33+.
Ellis, David. "The Defiant One." *People*, 19 December 1994, 46+.
Ferrel, Carolyn. "Don't Erase Me." *Don't Erase Me: Stories*. Boston: Houghton Mifflin, 1997. 39–67.
Fierstein, Harvey. "On Tidy Endings." *Safe Sex*. New York: Atheneum, 1987.
Fisher, Mary. *I'll Not Go Quietly: Mary Fisher Speaks Out*. New York: Scribner, 1995.
———. *Sleep with the Angels: A Mother Challenges AIDS*. Wakefield, Rhode Island: Moyer Bell, 1994.
Glaser, Elizabeth, and Laura Palmer. *In the Absence of Angels: A Hollywood Family's Courageous Story*. New York: Putnam, 1991.
Hambly, Barbara. *Fever Season*. New York: Bantam, 1999.
Harper, Frances E. W. *Iola Leroy*. 1893. Boston: Beacon, 1987.

Hawthorne, Nathaniel. "Lady Eleanor's Mantle." *Hawthorne: Tales and Sketches.* Literary Classics of the United States. New York: Viking, 1982. 652–66.

Hoffman, Alice. *At Risk.* New York: Berkley, 1988.

Jacobs, Harriet. *Incidents in the Life of a Slave Girl.* Ed. Jean Fagin Yellin. Cambridge: Harvard University Press, 1987.

Jezebel. Dir. William Wyler. Perf. Henry Fonda, Bette Davis, George Brent, Theresa Harris, and Eddie Anderson. Warner Brothers, 1938.

Klass, Perri. *Baby Doctor: A Pediatrician's Training.* New York: Random House, 1992.

———. *Other Women's Children.* New York: Random House, 1990.

Kushner, Tony. *Angels in America—Part One: Millennium Approaches.* New York: Theatre Communications Group, 1993.

———. *Angels in America—Part Two: Perestroika.* New York: Theatre Communications Group, 1994.

Larsen, Nella. *Quicksand and Passing.* New Brunswick, N.J.: Rutgers University Press, 1986.

"Leona's Sister, Gerri." Prod. and dir. Jane Gillooly. *POV.* WNET, New York. 3 November 1995.

Marvin's Room. Dir. Jerry Zaks. Perf. Meryl Streep, Diane Keaton, Leonardo DiCaprio, Hume Cronyn, and Robert DeNiro. Tribeca Productions, 1996.

Monette, Paul. *Halfway Home.* New York: Crown, 1991.

Morrison, Toni. *Beloved.* New York: Knopf, 1987.

Neely, Barbara. *Blanche on the Lam.* New York: Penguin, 1992.

O'Neill, Eugene. *The Complete Plays.* Literary Classics of the United States. New York: Viking, 1988.

Philadelphia. Dir. Jonathan Demme. Perf. Tom Hanks, Denzel Washington, Jason Robards, Antonio Banderas, and Mary Steenburgen. TriStar Pictures, 1993.

A Place for Annie. Dir. John Gray. Perf. Sissy Spacek, Mary-Louise Parker, and Joan Plowright. Hallmark Hall of Fame. ABC. WABC, New York. 1 May 1994.

Porter, Katherine Anne. "Pale Horse, Pale Rider." *Pale Horse, Pale Rider: Three Short Novels.* New York: Signet Modern Classic, 1962. 113–65.

Quindlen, Anna. *One True Thing.* New York: Dell, 1994.

Rudd, Andrea, and Darien Taylor, eds. *Positive Women: Voices of Women Living with AIDS.* Toronto: Second Story, 1992.

Sapphire. *Push.* New York: Knopf, 1996.

Selah, Tiye Milan. "An Elegy for Jade." In *Sisterfire: Black Womanist Fiction and Poetry,* ed. Charlotte Watson Sherman. New York: HarperCollins, 1994. 113–22.

Sherman, Charlotte Watson, ed. *Sisterfire: Black Womanist Fiction and Poetry.* New York: HarperCollins, 1994.

———. *touch.* New York: HarperCollins, 1995.

Stepmom. Dir. Chris Columbus. Perf. Susan Sarandon, Julia Roberts, and Ed Harris. TriStar Pictures, 1998.

Stowe, Harriet Beecher. *Uncle Tom's Cabin or, Life among the Lowly.* 1852. New York: Penguin, 1981.

Warner, Susan. *The Wide, Wide, World.* 1851. New York: Feminist, 1987.

II. Secondary Sources

ACT UP/NY Women and AIDS Book Group. *Women, AIDS and Activism.* Boston: South End, 1990.

Adams, Margaret. "The Compassion Trap." In *Woman in Sexist Society: Studies in Power and Powerlessness*, ed. Vivian Gornick and Barbara K. Moran. New York: New American Library, 1972. 555–75.

"Affordable Drug Reduces Mother-to-Child HIV Transmission, Study Says." *CNN Interactive* 14 July 1999. 14 July 1999. <http://www.cnn.com/HEALTH/AIDS/9907/14/preventing.baby.hiv/index.html>.

Allison, Dorothy. "A Question of Class." *Skin: Talking about Sex, Class and Literature*. Ithaca: Firebrand, 1994. 13–36.

Als, Hilton. *The Women*. New York: Farrar Straus Giroux, 1996.

Ammons, Elizabeth. "Stowe's Dream of the Mother-Savior: *Uncle Tom's Cabin* and American Women Writers before the 1920s." In *New Essays on Uncle Tom's Cabin*, ed. Eric J. Sundquist. New York: Cambridge University Press, 1986. 155–95.

Anastos, Kathryn, M.D., and Carola Marte, M.D. "Women—The Missing Persons in the AIDS Epidemic." *Health/PAC Bulletin* (winter 1989): 6–13.

Ards, Angela. "The New Black Radicalism." *Nation*, 27 July/3 August 1998, 19–23.

Arno, Peter S., Carol Levine, and Margaret M. Memmot. "The Economic Value of Informal Caregiving." *Health Affairs* 18, no.2 (1999): 182–88.

Averit, Dawn. "New Studies Show Why Research on Women Is Needed." *World*, August 1997, 4–6.

Bailey, Ruby L. "Sapphire's Dark Tale Is a Diamond in the Rough." *Detroit News*, 22 July 1996, B1.

Baker, Rob. *The Art of AIDS*. New York: Continuum, 1994.

Bates, Barbara. *Bargaining for Life: A Social History of Tuberculosis, 1876–1938*. Philadelphia: University of Pennsylvania Press, 1992.

Bawer, Bruce. "Hail Mary." *Advocate*, 25 July 1995, 63–64.

Baym, Nina. *Woman's Fiction: A Guide to Novels by and about Women in America, 1820–1870*. Ithaca: Cornell University Press, 1978.

Bell-Scott, Patricia. "The Artist as Witness: A Conversation with Sapphire." Rev. of *Push* by Sapphire. *Ms.* 7, no. 5 (March/April 1997): 78–81.

Berer, Marge, with Sunanda Ray. *Women and AIDS: An International Resource Book*. London: Pandora, 1993.

Berlant, Lauren. "Poor Eliza." *American Literature* 70, no. 3 (September 1998): 635–68.

Bethea, Plyshette Y. "Recent Studies Show Gender Difference in HIV-1 Viral Loads." *New Jersey Women and AIDS Network News*, spring 1999, 4.

Blaxton, Reginald Glenn. " 'Jesus Wept': Reflections on HIV Dis-ease and the Churches of Black Folk." In *Dangerous Liaisons: Blacks, Gays, and the Struggle for Equality*, ed. Eric Brandt. New York: New Press, 1999. 102–41.

Bobo, Jacqueline. "*The Color Purple*: Black Women as Cultural Readers." In *Women, Culture, and Society: A Reader*, ed. Barbara Balliet, with Susana Fried. Dubuque: Kendall/Hunt, 1992. 253–67.

Bogle, Donald. *Toms, Coons, Mulattoes, Mammies and Bucks: An Interpretive History of Blacks in American Films*. New York: Viking, 1994.

Bojar, Karen. "RE: Welfare reform outcomes" "Let Them Scrub Floors." On-line posting. Women's Studies List. 5 May 2000 <WMST-L@UMDD.UMD.EDU>.

Boykin, Keith. *One More River to Cross: Black and Gay in America*. New York: Doubleday, 1996.

Brownmiller, Susan. *Femininity*. London: Paladin, 1986.

Brownworth, Victoria A. "Someone Has to Say No: Women in Gay Male Writing." *Lambda Book Report*, October/November 1990, 6+.

Burkett, Elinor. *The Gravest Show on Earth: America in the Age of AIDS*. New York: Houghton Mifflin, 1995.

Byrne, Hugh. Letter. *Irish Voice,* 9–15 July 1997, 13.

Cady, Joseph. "Teaching about AIDS through Literature in a Medical School Curriculum." In *Confronting AIDS through Literature: The Responsibilities of Representation,* ed. Judith Laurence Pastore. Urbana: University of Illinois Press, 1993. 233–48.

Carby, Hazel V. *Reconstructing Womanhood: The Emergence of the Afro-American Woman Novelist.* New York: Oxford University Press, 1987.

Carovano, Kathryn. "More Than Mothers and Whores: Redefining the AIDS Prevention Needs of Women." *International Journal of Health Services* 21, no. 1 (1991): 131–42.

Case, Sue-Ellen. "Toward a Butch-Feminist Retro-Future." In *Cross Purposes: Lesbians, Feminists, and the Limits of Alliance,* ed. Dana Heller. Bloomington: Indiana University Press, 1997. 205–220.

Cherniavsky, Eva. *That Pale Mother Rising: Sentimental Discourses and the Imitation of Motherhood in Nineteenth-Century America.* Bloomington: Indiana University Press, 1995.

Clarke, Cheryl. "An Identity of One's Own." *Harvard Gay and Lesbian Review* (fall 1996): 37–38.

Cohen, Cathy J. *The Boundaries of Blackness: AIDS and the Breakdown of Blacks Politics.* Chicago: University of Chicago Press, 1999.

Cohen, Cathy, and Tamara Jones. "Fighting Homophobia versus Challenging Heterosexism: 'The Failure to Transform' Revisited." In *Dangerous Liaisons: Blacks, Gays, and the Struggle for Equality,* ed. Eric Brandt. New York: New Press, 1999. 80–101.

Collette, Ann. "Damm, She Done It: Barbara Neely's Fictional Detective Fights More Than Crime." *Ms.,* June/July 2000, 77–79.

Collins, Patricia Hill. "Mammies, Matriarchs, and Other Controlling Images." *Black Feminist Thought: Knowledge, Consciousness, and the Politics of Empowerment.* New York: Routledge, 1991. 67–90.

——. "Black Women and Motherhood." In *Rereading America: Cultural Contexts for Critical Thinking and Writing,* ed. Gary Colombo, Robert Cullen, and Bonnie Lisle. Boston: Bedford, 1995. 195–211.

"A Conversation with Donna Haraway: 'More Than You Think, Less Than There Should Be.' " *Praxis* (1991): 1–21.

Corea, Gena. *The Invisible Epidemic: Story of Women and AIDS.* New York: HarperCollins, 1992.

Corliss, Richard. "Family Therapy: *Marvin's Room.*" *Time,* 30 December 1996, 159.

Cott, Nancy. *The Bonds of Womanhood: "Woman's Sphere" in New England, 1780–1835.* New Haven: Yale University Press, 1977.

Crimp, Douglas. *AIDS: Cultural Analysis, Cultural Activism.* Cambridge: MIT Press, 1988.

——. "How to Have Promiscuity during an Epidemic." In *AIDS: Cultural Analysis, Cultural Activism,* ed. Crimp. Cambridge: MIT Press, 1988. 237–271.

——. "Mourning and Militancy." *October* 51 (winter 1989): 1–18.

Cvetkovich, Ann. *Mixed Feelings: Feminism, Mass Culture, and Victorian Sensationalism.* New Brunswick, N.J.: Rutgers University Press, 1992.

Danica, Elly. *Don't: A Woman's Word, A Personal Chronicle of Childhood Incest and Adult Recovery.* Pittsburgh: Cleis, 1988.

Davidson, Cathy N., and Linda Wagner-Martin. *The Oxford Companion to Women's Writing in the United States.* New York: Oxford University Press, 1995.

Davis, Angela. "Defending Our Name." *Sojourner: The Women's Forum* 19, no. 11 (July 1994): 1.

DeLombard, Jeannine. "Who Cares? Lesbians as Caregivers." In *Dyke Life: From Growing Up to Growing Old*, ed. Karla Jay. New York: Basic Books, 1995. 344–61.

Denenberg, Risa, FNP. "Positive Lesbians Deserve the Best!" *LAP Notes: Lesbian AIDS Project at GMHC* 5 (1997): 1.

Denison, Rebecca. "Call Us Survivors! Women Organized to Respond to Life Threatening Diseases (WORLD)." In *Women Resisting AIDS: Strategies of Empowerment*, ed. Beth E. Schneider and Nancy E. Stoller. Philadelphia: Temple University Press, 1995. 195–207.

——. "AIDS Death Decline for Men, but Increase for Women." *World*, April 1997, 1.

——. "Pediatric AIDS Update." *World*, June 1997, 5.

——. "New Guidelines for Use of HIV Drugs during Pregnancy." *World*, April 1998, 4–6

——. "Proud to Be a Lab Rat." *World*, July 1998, 4–5.

——. "Pregnancy and Perinatal Transmission Update." *World*, September 1998, 6–7.

——. "Understanding HIV and AIDS: The Basics." *World*, June 2000, 4.

——. "Women and AIDS: An Update." *World*, May 1997, 4–7.

Denneny, Michael. "AIDS Writing and the Creation of a Gay Culture." In *Confronting AIDS through Literature: The Responsibilities of Representation*, ed. Judith Laurence Pastore. Urbana: University of Illinois Press, 1993. 36–54.

Deprez, Luisa S. "Classist Conceptions of Dependency: Conservative Attacks on Poor Women with Children." In *Speaking Out: Women, Poverty, and Public Policy: Proceedings of the Twenty-Third Annual Women's Studies Conference, University of Wisconsin System Women's Studies Consortium, 29–31 October 1998*, ed. Katherine A. Rhoades and Anne Statham. 25 May 2000. <http://www.library.wisc.edu/libraries/WomensStudies/othsubj.htm#WELFARE>.

"Determination Marks Opening of Third National Conference on Women and HIV." *PRNewswire*. On-line. Channel Q News Service. 5 May 1997.

Dewey, Joseph. "Music for a Closing: Responses to AIDS in Three American Novels." In *AIDS: The Literary Response*, ed. Emmanuel S. Nelson. New York: Twayne, 1992. 23–38.

Diaz, Marlene, and Rebecca Denison. "What We Learned the Hard Way." *World*, March 1997, 6.

DiQuinzio, Patrice. *The Impossibility of Motherhood: Feminism, Individualism, and the Problem of Mothering*. New York & London: Routledge, 1999.

Douglas, Ann. *The Feminization of American Culture*. New York: Knopf, 1977.

——. Introduction. *Uncle Tom's Cabin or, Life among the Lowly*, by Harriet Beecher Stowe. New York: Penguin, 1981. 7–34.

Douglas, Susan. "The Mommy Wars." *Ms.* 10, no. 2 (February/March 2000): 62–68.

Ducksworth, Sarah Smith. In *The Stowe Debate: Rhetorical Strategies in Uncle Tom's Cabin*, ed. Mason I. Lowance, Jr., Ellen E. Westbrook, and R.C. De Prospo. Amherst: U of Massachusetts P, 1994. 205–235.

Ebert, Roger. Rev. of *Marvin's Room*. *Chicago Sun-Times*, 11 January 1997, 14 July 1998. <http://www.suntimes.com/ebert/ebert_reviews/1997/01/011002.html>.

Erni, John Nguyet. Personal communication to author. January 2000.

Faderman, Lillian. Afterword. In *Cross Purposes: Lesbians, Feminists, and the Limits of Alliance*, ed. Dana Heller. Bloomington: Indiana University Press, 1997. 221–29.

——. *Odd Girls and Twilight Lovers: A History of Lesbian Life in Twentieth-Century America*. New York: Penguin, 1991.

Farber, Celia. "AZT Roulette: The Impossible Choices Facing HIV-Positive Women." *Mothering*, September–October 1998, 53–65.

Feehan, Amy. "Expecting the Worst: One Thing Gets Policymakers Interested in the Lives of Women with HIV—Pregnancy." *POZ*, August–September 1995, 54+.

Ferguson, Kathy E. "Writing 'Kibbutz Journal': Borders, Voices, and the Traffic in Between." In *Talking Gender: Public Images, Personal Journeys, and Political Critiques*, ed. Nancy Hewitt, Jean O'Barr, and Nancy Rosebaugh. Chapel Hill: University of North Carolina Press, 1996. 84–105.

Fine, Gary Allen. "Welcome to the World of AIDS: Fantasies of Women's Revenge." *Western Folklore* 46 (1987): 192–97.

Fitzpatrick, Laurie. "Voice of the People." *A&U*, July 1997, 30–37.

France, David. "A Dangerous Women." *Mirabella*, April 1995, 96–100.

Francis, Lynde. "Breastfeeding Prospective: African Women Need Choices." *WORLD: Women Organized to Respond to Life-Threatening Diseases: A Newsletter by, for, and about Women Facing HIV Disease*, September 1998, 5.

Franzen, Jonathan. "Hitting the Road." Rev. of *Bone*, by Russell Banks. *New York Times Book Review*, 7 May 1996, 1+.

Gamble, Vanessa Northington. "No Medical Miracles." *Women's Review of Books* VIII, no. 3 (December 1990): 10–11.

Gates, Henry Louis. Introduction. *Reading Black, Reading Feminist: A Critical Anthology*, ed Gates. New York: Meridian, 1990. 1–25.

Golden, Stephanie. *Slaying the Mermaid: Women and the Culture of Sacrifice*. New York: Harmony Books, 1998.

Gomez, Jewelle. Rev. of *Push* by Sapphire. *Ms.* 7, no. 5 (July/August 1996): 82.

Gorna, Robin. *Vamps, Virgins, and Victims: How Can Women Fight AIDS?* London: Cassell, 1996.

Grey, Amanda. "The Right Kind of Push." Rev. of *Push* by Sapphire. *New Youth Connections*, September/October 1996, 19.

Groeger, Anne. "Women and AIDS: Get the Facts!" *WORLD: Women Organized to Respond to Life-Threatening Diseases: A Newsletter by, for, and about Women Facing HIV Disease* 56 (December 1995): 4–5.

Guthmann, Edward. "This Is a 'Room' Full of Acting." *San Francisco Chronicle*, 10 January 1997, D3.

Hamburger, Aaron. "Boxed In." *New York Blade News*, 15 May 1998, 21, 23.

Hammonds, Evelynn. "Black (W)holes and the Geometry of Black Female Sexuality." *differences* 6, nos. 2–3 (1994): 126–45.

———. "Missing Persons: African American Women, AIDS, and the History of Disease." *Radical America*, July 1992, 7–23.

———. "Race, Sex, AIDS: The Construction of 'Other.' " *Radical America*, September 1987, 28–36.

———. "Seeing AIDS: Race, Gender, and Representation." In *The Gender Politics of HIV/AIDS in Women: Perspectives on the Pandemic in the United States*, ed. Nancy Goldstein and Jennifer L. Manlowe. New York: New York University Press, 1997. 113–26.

Hansen, Eileen. "No Mandatory HIV Testing! No Mandatory AZT for Pregnant Women!" *World*, August 1995, 3.

Hanson, Ellis. Introduction. In *Outtakes: Essays on Queer Theory and Film*, ed. Hanson. Durham & London: Duke University Press, 1999. 1–19.

Hardy, James Earl. "Personal Hits." *Advocate*, 24 June 1997, 104.

Harper, Marques. "Spread Awareness to Campus." *Daily Targum*, 5 May 1997, 14–15.

Harrington, Imani. "American Quarantine: Isolation, Alienation, Deprivation." In *Positive Women: Voices of Women Living with AIDS*, ed. Andrea Rudd and Darien Taylor. Toronto: Second Story, 1992. 178–86.

Harrington, Susanmarie. "Women and AIDS: Bodily Representations, Political Repercussions." In *Bodily Discursions: Genders, Representations, Technologies*, ed. Deborah S. Wilson and Christine Moneera Laennec. Albany: State University of New York Press, 1997. 201–20.

Harris, Trudier. *From Mammies to Militants: Domestics in Black Literature*. Philadelphia: Temple University Press, 1982.

Hartman, Stephanie. E-mail to author. 15 March 1996.

Hewitt, Nancy A. "Beyond the Search for Sisterhood: American Women's History in the 1980s." In *Unequal Sisters: A Multicultural Reader in U.S. Women's History*, ed. Carol Ellen DuBois and Vicki L. Ruiz. New York: Routledge, 1990. 1–14.

Holland, Janet, Caroline Ramazanoglu, Sue Scott, and Rachel Thomson. "Power and Desire: The Embodiment of Female Sexuality." *Feminist Review* 46 (spring 1994): 21–38.

Hood, Carra Leah. "Scarlett Begat Kim: A Counter-Biography." In *Gendered Epidemic: Representations of Women in the Age of AIDS*, ed. Nancy L. Roth and Katie Hogan. New York: Routledge, 1998. 153–64.

hooks, bell. "Ain't She Still a Woman?" *BRC-NEWS* 12 December 1999.

——. *Black Looks: Race and Representation*. Boston: South End, 1992.

——. *Reel to Real: Race, Sex, and Class at the Movies*. New York: Routledge, 1996.

——. *Teaching to Transgress*. New York: Routledge, 1994.

——. *Yearning: Race, Gender, and Cultural Politics*. Boston: South End, 1991.

Horvath, Hacsi. "Women and AIDS: The Forgotten Epidemic." *CNN Interactive* 9 July 1999. 14 July 1999 <http://www.cnn.com/HEALTH/AIDS/9907/09/women.aids>.

Huston, River, and Mary Berridge. *A Positive Life: Portraits of Women Living with HIV*. Philadelphia: Running Press, 1997.

Ian, Marcia. Personal communication to author. August 1993–August 1997.

James, Caryn. "*At Risk* Author Discusses Fears about AIDS." *New York Times*, 18 July 1988, C15.

Johnson, Deborah. "Women Who Trust Too Much: What AIDS Commercials Don't Tell You." *On the Issues: The Progressive Woman's Quarterly* 5, no. 3 (summer 1996): 26–28.

Jordan, June. *Technical Difficulties: African-American Notes on the State of the Union*. New York: Villard, 1994.

Juhasz, Alexandra. "The Contained Threat: Women in Mainstream AIDS Documentary." *Journal of Sex Research* 27, no. 1 (February 1990): 25–46.

Kachuck, Beatrice. "Re: A Great Project." On-line posting. Women's Studies List. 17 July 1997. <WMST-L@UMDD.UMD.EDU>.

Kahn, Peggy, et al. "Work Requirements and the Care Crisis: Everyday Lives of Single Welfare Mothers under the New Welfare Laws." In *Speaking Out: Women, Poverty, and Public Policy: Proceedings of the Twenty-Third Annual Women's Studies Conference, University of Wisconsin System Women's Studies Consortium, 29–31 October 1998*, ed. Katherine A. Rhoades and Anne Statham. 25 May 2000. <http://www.library.wisc.edu/libraries/WomensStudies/othsubj.htm#WELFARE>.

Keeley, Carol. "Women on the Verge: The Needs of HIV Positive Women Are Not Being Addressed." *POZ*, August–September 1995, 50+.

Keniston, Kenneth. "Introduction to the Issue." In *Living with AIDS*, ed. Stephen R. Graubard. Cambridge: MIT Press, 1990.

Kennedy, Lisa. "Shoved." Rev. of *Push*, by Sapphire. *Village Voice*, 25 June 1996, 76.

Kerber, Linda K. "Separate Spheres, Female Worlds, Woman's Place: The Rhetoric of Women's History." *Journal of American History* 75 (June 1988): 9–39.

Kimoto, Diane M. "Affirming Role of Women as Carers: The Social Construction of AIDS through the Eyes of Mother, Friend, and Nurse." In *Women and AIDS: Negotiating Safer Practices, Care, and Representation*, ed. Nancy L. Roth and Linda K. Fuller. New York: Harrington Park, 1998. 155–79.

Kitzinger, Jenny. "Visible and Invisible Women in AIDS Discourse." In *AIDS: Setting a Feminist Agenda*, ed. Lesley Doyal, Jennie Naidoo, and Tamsin Wilton. London: Taylor & Francis, 1994. 95–112.

Koelsch, Patrice Clark. "Mortal Combats." Rev. of *How to Have Theory in an Epidemic*, by Paula Treichler. *Women's Review of Books*, March 2000, 18–20.

Koonz, Claudia. *Mothers in the Fatherland: Women, the Family and Nazi Politics*. New York: St. Martin's, 1987.

Krieg, Joann P. *Epidemics in the Modern World*. New York: Twayne, 1992.

Kruger, Steven F. *AIDS Narratives: Gender and Sexuality, Fiction and Science*. New York: Garland, 1996.

Ladonna. "Listen to Children . . . They're Great Teachers." *World*, March 1997, 1–2.

Leavitt, David. "The Way I Live Now." *New York Times Magazine*, 9 July 1988, 28.

Levine, Carol. "The Loneliness of the Long-Term Care Giver." *New England Journal of Medicine* 340, no. 2 (May 1999): 1587–90.

Lipsitz, George. "The Greatest Story Ever Sold: Marketing and the O. J. Simpson Trial." In *Birth of a Nation 'hood: Gaze, Script, and Spectacle in the O. J. Simpson Case*, ed. Toni Morrison and Claudia Brodsky Lacour. New York: Pantheon, 1997. 3–29.

Liss, Andrea. "The Body in Question: Rethinking Motherhood, Alterity and Desire." In *New Feminist Criticism: Art, Identity, Action*, ed. Joanna Frueh, Cassandra L. Langer, and Arlene Raven. New York: HarperCollins, 1994. 80–96.

Long, Lynellyn D., and E. Maxine Ankrah. *Women's Experiences with HIV/AIDS: An International Perspective*. New York: Columbia University Press, 1996.

Lorber, Judith. *Paradoxes of Gender*. New Haven: Yale University Press, 1994.

Lubiano, Wahneema. "Black Ladies, Welfare Queens, and State Minstrels: Ideological Warfare by Narrative Means." In *Race-ing Justice, En-gendering Power: Essays on Anita Hill, Clarence Thomas, and the Construction of Social Reality*, ed. Toni Morrison. New York: Pantheon, 1992. 323–361.

MacFarlene, Lisa Watt. "Harriet Beecher Stowe." In *The Oxford Companion to Women's Writing in the United States*, ed. Cathy N. Davidson and Linda Wagner-Martin. New York: Oxford University Press, 1995. 856–58.

Maldonado, Miguelina. "State of Emergency: HIV/AIDS among African Americans." *National Minority AIDS Council Update*, September 1998, 1–12.

Manring, M. M. *Slave in a Box: The Strange Career of Aunt Jemima*. Charlottesville: University Press of Virginia, 1998.

Marshall, Stuart. "Picturing Deviancy." In *Ecstatic Antibodies: Resisting the AIDS Mythology*, ed. Tessa Boffin and Sunil Gupta. London: Rivers Oram, 1990. 19–36.

Martinac, Paula. "Lesbian Notions." *EXP Magazine*, 29 July–4 August 1998, 34.

Maslin, Janet. "Another Buddy Story, with a Twist or Two." Rev. of *Boys on the Side*, dir. Herbert Ross. *New York Times*, 3 February 1995, C3.

——. "Bittersweet Lessons as a Family Reunites." Rev. of *Marvin's Room*. *New York Times*, 18 December 1996, C15.

McAllister, Linda Lopez. Review of *Marvin's Room*. *The Woman's Show*. WMNF, Tampa. 1 March 1997.

McCallum, Heather. "The Ideological Foundations of the TANF Welfare Rules." In *Speaking Out: Women, Poverty, and Public Policy: Proceedings of the Twenty-Third Annual Women's Studies Conference, University of Wisconsin System Women's Studies Consortium, 29–31 October 1998*, ed. Katherine A. Rhoades and Anne Statham. 25 May 2000. <http://www.library.wisc.edu/libraries/WomensStudies/othsubj.htm#WELFARE>.

McCaskill, Barbara, and Layli Phillips. "We Are All 'Good Woman!': A Womanist Critique of the Current Feminist Conflict." In *Bad Girls/Good Girls: Women, Sex, and Power in the Nineties*, ed. Nan Bauer Maglin and Donna Perry. New Brunswick, N.J.: Rutgers University Press, 1996. 106–22.

Miller, James, ed. *Fluid Exchanges: Artists and Critics in the AIDS Crisis*. Toronto: University of Toronto Press, 1992.

Milton, Edith. "Fantasies of Suburbia." Rev. of *At Risk*, by Alice Hoffman. *Women's Review of Books*, December 1990, 17–18.

Mink, Gwendolyn. "The Lady and the Tramp: Gender, Race, and the Origins of the American Welfare State." In *Women, Culture, and Society: A Reader*, ed. Barbara Balliet, with Susana Fried. Dubuque: Kendall/Hunt, 1992. 371–92.

Modleski, Tania. "In Hollywood, Racist Stereotypes Can Still Earn Oscar Nominations." *Chronicle of Higher Education* 17 (March 2000): B9.

———. *Loving with a Vengeance: Mass-Produced Fantasies for Women*. London: Methuen, 1982.

Mullen, Harryette. "Runaway Tongue: Resistant Orality in *Uncle Tom's Cabin, Our Nig, Incidents in the Life of a Slave Girl*, and *Beloved*." In *The Culture of Sentiment: Race, Gender, and Sentimentality in 19th Century America*, ed. Shirley Samuels. New York: Oxford UP, 1992. 244–264.

Mulvey, Laura. "Visual Pleasure and Narrative Cinema." *Screen* 16 (1975): 6–18.

Murphy, Timothy F. "The Angry Death of Kimberly Bergalis." *Ethics in an Epidemic: AIDS, Morality, and Culture*. Berkeley: University of California Press, 1994.

Murray, Charles. "Keeping Priorities Straight on Welfare Reform." *Society* 33, no. 5 (July–August 1996): 10–13.

Nelson, Emmanuel S., ed. *AIDS: The Literary Response*. New York: Twayne, 1992.

New Jersey Women and AIDS Network News. 1990–.

Ngcobo, Lauretta. "African Motherhood: Fact and Fiction." In *Critical Fictions: The Politics of Imaginative Writing*, ed. Philimina Mariani. Seattle: Bay, 1991. 194–99.

Nuernberg, Susan Marie. In *The Stowe Debate: Rhetorical Strategies in Uncle Tom's Cabin*, ed. Mason I. Lowance, Jr., Ellen E. Westbrook, and R.C. De Prospo. Amherst: U of Massachusetts P, 1994. 255–270.

O'Connell, Catharine E. " 'The Magic of the Real Presence of Distress': Sentimentality and Competing Rhetorics of Authority." In *The Stowe Debate: Rhetorical Strategies in Uncle Tom's Cabin*, ed. Mason I. Lowance Jr., Ellen E. Westbrook, and R. C. De Prospo. Amherst: University of Massachusetts Press, 1994. 13–36.

Odets Walt. *In the Shadow of the Epidemic: Being HIV Negative in the Age of AIDS*. Durham, N.C.: Duke University Press, 1995.

O'Grady, Lorraine. "Olympia's Maid: Reclaiming Black Female Subjectivity." In *New Feminist Criticism: Art, Identity, Action*, ed. Joanna Frueh, Cassandra L. Langer, and Arlene Raven. New York: HarperCollins, 1994. 152–70.

Ogur, Barbara. "Smothering in Stereotypes: HIV-Positive Women." In *Talking Gender: Public Images, Personal Journeys, and Political Critiques*, ed. Nancy Hewitt, Jean O'Barr, and Nancy Rosebaugh. Chapel Hill: University of North Carolina Press, 1996. 137–52.

Parini, Jay. "Literary Theory Is Not All Bad." *Chronicle of Higher Education*, 17 November 1995, A52.

Park, Katharine. "Kimberly Bergalis, AIDS, and the Plague Metaphor." In *Media Spectacle*, ed. Marjorie Garber, Jann Matlock, and Rebbeca L. Walkowitz. New York: Routledge, 1993. 232–53.

Pastore, Judith Laurence. "Suburban AIDS: Alice Hoffman's *At Risk*." In *AIDS: The Literary Response*, ed. Emmanuel S. Nelson. New York: Twayne, 1992. 39–49.

Patton, Cindy. *Last Served? Gendering the HIV Pandemic*. London: Taylor & Francis, 1994.

Pemberton, Gayle. "Hello, Stranger." In *Skin Deep: Black and White Women Write about Race*, ed. Marita Golden and Susan Richards Shreve. New York: Anchor, 1995. 271–86.

Pincus, Elizabeth. "Side Dish." Rev. of *Boys on the Side*, dir. Herbert Ross. *Gay Community News*, winter 1995, 25–26.

Piontek, Thomas. "Unsafe Representations: Cultural Criticism in the Age of AIDS." *Discourse* 15, no. 1 (1992): 128–53.

Poovey, Mary. *Uneven Developments: The Ideological Work of Gender in Mid-Victorian England*. Chicago: University of Chicago Press, 1988.

Radford, Jean, ed. *The Progress of Romance: The Politics of Popular Fiction*. London: Routledge & Kegan Paul, 1986.

Radway, Janice A. *Reading the Romance: Women, Patriarchy, and Popular Literature*. Chapel Hill: University of North Carolina Press, 1984.

Rando, Flavia. "The Body, the Feminine, and the Names Project Memorial Quilt." In *Gendered Epidemic: Representations of Women in the Age of AIDS*, ed. Nancy L. Roth and Katie Hogan. New York: Routledge, 1998. 191–204.

Rapping, Elayne. "You've Come Which Way, Baby?" *Women's Review of Books*, July 2000, 20–22.

Reagan, Patty. Rev. of *Women and HIV/AIDS: An International Resource Book; Women and AIDS—Psychological Perspectives;* and *Until the Cure: Caring for Women with HIV*. *NWSA Journal* 7, no. 1 (spring 1995): 152–55.

Richardson, Diane. *Women and AIDS*. New York: Routledge, 1988.

Rieder, Ines, and Patricia Ruppelt, eds. *AIDS: The Women*. San Francisco: Cleis, 1988.

Rimer, Sara. "Group of Leading Blacks Urges Campaign on AIDS Awareness." *New York Times*, 25 October 1996, 18.

Roberson, Susan L. "Matriarchy and the Rhetoric of Domesticity." In *The Stowe Debate: Rhetorical Strategies in Uncle Tom's Cabin*, ed. Mason I. Lowance Jr., Ellen E. Westbrook, and R. C. De Prospo. Amherst: University of Massachusetts Press, 1994. 116–37.

Rorty, Richard. "The Necessity of Inspired Reading." *Chronicle of Higher Education*, 9 February 1996, A48.

Rosenfelt, Deborah Silverton. "Commentary." In *Salt of the Earth*, a screenplay by Michael Wilson. New York: Feminist Press, 1978. 93–168.

Rothman, Sheila M. *Living in the Shadow of Death: Tuberculosis and the Social Experience of Illness in American History*. New York: BasicBooks, 1994.

Rubinstein, Arye, et al. "Acquired Immunodeficiency with Reversed T4/T6 Ratios in Infants Born to Promiscuous and Drug-Addicted Mothers." *JAMA* 249, no. 17 (1983): 2350–56.

Rudd, Andrea, and Darien Taylor, eds. *Positive Women: Voices of Women Living with AIDS*. Toronto: Second Story, 1992.

Runions, Debbie. "HIV/AIDS: A Personal Perspective." In *Women's Experiences with HIV/AIDS: An International Perspective,* ed. Lynellyn D. Long and E. Maxine Ankrah. New York: Columbia University Press, 1996. 56–72.

Samuels, Shirley, ed. *The Culture of Sentiment: Race, Gender, and Sentimentality in Nineteenth-Century America.* New York: Oxford University Press, 1992.

Savran, David. "Ambivalence, Utopia, and a Queer Sort of Materialism: How *Angels in America* Reconstructs the Nation." *Theatre Journal* 47 (1995): 207–27.

Schilling, Carol. Rev. of *Confronting AIDS through Literature: The Responsibilities of Representation. Modern Language Studies* 24, no. 3 (1994): 110–12.

Schoofs, Mark. "Black Up! : African Americans Confront Their Worst Health Crisis: AIDS." *Village Voice,* 5 November 1996, 45.

——. "The Deadly Gender Gap." *Village Voice,* 5 January 1999, 33–34, 38.

——. "Death and the Second Sex." AIDS: The Agony of Africa, Part 5. *Village Voice,* 7 December 1999, 67+.

Schulman, Sarah. *Stagestruck: Theater, AIDS, and the Marketing of Gay America.* Durham: Duke University Press, 1998.

Sedgwick, Eve Kosofsky. *Epistemology of the Closet.* Berkeley: University of California Press, 1990.

Segal, Lynne. "Lessons from the Past: Feminism, Sexual Politics, and the Challenge of AIDS." In *Taking Liberties: AIDS and Cultural Politics,* ed. Erica Carter and Simon Watney. London: Serpent's Tail, 1989. 133–45.

Shepard, Jim. "She Would Have Been Beautiful." *New York Times Book Review,* 17 July 1988, 7.

Shernoff, Michael, MSW. "Challenges and Dilemmas Regarding Protease Inhibitors." *Body Positive,* March 1997, 15–18.

Showalter, Elaine. *Sexual Anarchy: Gender and Culture at the Fin de Siècle.* New York: Penguin, 1990.

Shulgasser, Barbara. "Laugh, Cry, and Grow Old with *Marvin." San Francisco Examiner,* 10 January 1997, C3.

Singer, Linda. *Erotic Welfare: Sexual Theory and Politics in the Age of Epidemic.* New York: Routledge, 1993.

Siporen, Carol. "AIDS in Women—A Different Disease." *World,* January 1998, 6–7.

Smith, Stephanie A. "Sentimental Journey." *Women's Review of Books* 10, no. 10 (July 1993): 41–42.

Smith, Valerie. *Not Just Race, Not Just Gender: Black Feminist Readings.* New York: Routledge, 1998.

Smith-Rosenberg, Carroll. *Disorderly Conduct: Visions of Gender in Victorian America.* New York: Oxford University Press, 1986.

Sontag, Susan. *Illness as Metaphor* and *AIDS and Its Metaphors.* New York: Doubleday, 1989.

Spillers, Hortense. "Changing the Letter: The Yokes, the Jokes of Discourse, or Mrs. Stowe, Mr. Reed." In *Slavery and the Literary Imagination,* ed. Deborah E. McDowell and Arnold Rampersand. Baltimore: Johns Hopkins University Press, 1989.

Stanovsky, Derek. "Princess Diana, Mother Teresa, and the Value of Women's Work." *NWSA Journal* 11, no. 2 (1999): 146–51.

Stolberg, Sheryl Gay. "The Better Half Got the Worse End." *New York Times,* 20 July 1997, sec. 4, 1+.

Stoller, Nancy E. "Lesbian Involvement in the AIDS Epidemic: Changing Roles and Generational Differences." In *Women Resisting AIDS: Feminist Strategies of Empow-*

erment, ed. Beth E. Schneider and Nancy E. Stoller. Philadelphia: Temple University Press, 1995. 270–85.

Sullivan, Andrew. "When Plagues End: Notes on the Twilight of an Epidemic." *New York Times Magazine,* 10 November 1996, 52+.

Summers, Claude J., ed. *The Gay and Lesbian Literary Heritage: A Reader's Companion to the Writers and Their Works, from Antiquity to the Present.* New York: Henry Holt, 1995.

Taylor, Helen. "Gone With the Wind: The Mammy of Them All." In *The Progress of Romance: The Politics of Popular Fiction,* ed. Jean Radford. London: Routledge & Kegan Paul, 1986. 113–36.

Thielmann, Pia. "Black-White Love in African Novels." *Women's Studies Quarterly* 25, nos. 3, 4 (fall/winter 1997): 53–67.

Tobin, Nathan. "Disrobing the Welfare Queen." *AlterNet.org* 12 July 2000. <http://www.alternet.org/print.html?/StoryID=9435>.

——. "Disrobing the Welfare Queen." *AlterNet.org* 12 July 2000. 12 December 1999. <http://www.shambhalasun.com/Archives/Columnists/Hooks/HooksJan99.ht>

Tompkins, Jane. *Sensational Designs: The Cultural Work of American Fiction, 1790–1860.* New York: Oxford University Press, 1985.

Toner, Robin. "Pulling Strings: Invoking the Moral Authority of Moms." *New York Times,* 7 May 2000, 1+.

Treichler, Paula. "AIDS, Gender, and Biomedical Discourse: Current Contests for Meaning." In *AIDS: The Burdens of History,* ed. Elizabeth Fee and Daniel M. Fox. Berkeley: University of California Press, 1988. 190–226.

——. "AIDS, Homophobia, and Biomedical Discourse: An Epidemic of Signification." In *AIDS: Cultural Analysis, Cultural Activism,* ed. Douglas Crimp. Cambridge: MIT Press, 1988. 31–70.

——. "Beyond *Cosmo:* AIDS, Identity, and Inscriptions of Gender." *Camera Obscura* 28 (1992): 21–76.

——. *How to Have Theory in an Epidemic: Cultural Chronicles of AIDS.* Durham, N.C.: Duke University Press, 1999.

Turner, Patricia A. *Ceramic Uncles and Celluloid Mammies: Black Images and Their Influence on Culture.* New York: Anchor, 1994.

Update. National Minority AIDS Council. September 1998.

Vaidhyanathan, Siva. "Inside a 'Model Minority': The Complicated Identity of South Asians." *Chronicle of Higher Education,* 23 June 2000, B4.

Valian, Virginia. *Why So Slow? The Advancement of Women.* Cambridge: MIT Press, 1998.

Vance, Carole S., ed. *Pleasure and Danger: Exploring Female Sexuality.* Boston: Routledge & Kegan Paul, 1984.

Vassall, E. Rikki. "Sexual Assault and HIV." *WORLD: Women Organized to Respond to Life-Threatening Diseases: A Newsletter by, for, and about Women Facing HIV Disease,* June 1994, 2–5.

Vázquez, Carmen. Unpublished talk. Town meeting on HIV/AIDS prevention, Lesbian and Gay Community Services Center, New York City. 16 November 1994.

Wagner-Martin, Linda. *Telling Women's Lives: The New Biography.* New Brunswick, N.J.: Rutgers University Press, 1994. 15–18.

Walters, Suzanna Danuta. *Material Girls: Making Sense of Feminist Cultural Theory.* Berkeley: University of California Press, 1995.

Wardley, Lynn. "Relic, Fetish, Femmage: The Aesthetics of Sentiment in the Work of Stowe." In *The Culture of Sentiment: Race, Gender, and Sentimentality in Nineteenth-*

Century America, ed. Shirley Samuels. New York: Oxford University Press, 1992. 203–20.

Waugh. Thomas. "Erotic Self-Images in the Gay Male AIDS Melodrama." In *Fluid Exchanges: Artists and Critics in the AIDS Crisis*, ed. James Miller. Toronto: Toronto UP, 1992. 122–134.

Wexler, Laura. "Tender Violence: Literary Eavesdropping, Domestic Fiction, and Educational Reform." In *The Culture of Sentiment: Race, Gender, and Sentimentality in Nineteenth-Century America*, ed. Shirley Samuels. New York: Oxford University Press, 1992. 9–38.

White, Deborah Gray. *Arn't I a Woman? Female Slaves in the Plantation South*. New York: W. W. Norton, 1985.

——. "Private Lives, Public Personae: A Look at Early Twentieth-Century African American Clubwomen." In *Talking Gender: Public Images, Personal Journeys, and Political Critiques*, ed. Nancy Hewitt, Jean O'Barr, and Nancy Rosebaugh. Chapel Hill: University of North Carolina Press, 1996. 106–23.

White, E. Frances. "HMO Kills Baby: The Tabitha Walrond Case." On-line posting. Black Radical Congress Press. 24 June 1999. <http://www.egroups.com/group/brc-press>.

White, Isabelle. "Sentimentality and the Uses of Death." In *The Stowe Debate: Rhetorical Strategies in Uncle Tom's Cabin*, ed. Mason I. Lowance Jr., Ellen E. Westbrook, and R.C. De Prospo. Amherst: University of Massachusetts Press, 1994. 99–115.

Williamson, Judith. "Every Virus Tells a Story: The Meaning of HIV and AIDS." In *Taking Liberties: AIDS and Cultural Politics*, ed. Erica Carter and Simon Watney. London: Serpent's Tail, 1989. 69–80.

Wood, Julia T. *Who Cares? Women, Care, and Culture*. Carbondale: Southern Illinois University Press, 1994.

WORLD: Women Organized to Respond to Life-Threatening Diseases: A Newsletter by, for, and about Women Facing HIV Disease. May 1991–.

Zimmer, Elizabeth. "Angel in Brooklyn." Rev. of *The Whispers of Angels*, chor. David Rousseve. Brooklyn Academy of Music. Majestic Theater, New York. *Village Voice*, 5 December 1995, 34.

Zook, Kristal Brent. "A Manifesto of Sorts for a Black Feminist Movement." *New York Times Magazine*, 12 November 1995, 86+.

INDEX

ABOUT THE AUTHOR

Katie Hogan is an associate professor of English at LaGuardia Community College, City University of New York. She is the editor, with Nancy L. Roth, of *Gendered Epidemic: Representations of Women in the Age of AIDS* (Routledge, 1998). She was the recipient of the 1996 Pergamon-National Women's Studies Association Award for Graduate Scholarship in Women's Studies and of a 1999 CUNY Research Foundation Award.